An Evaluation of Policy-Related Rehabilitation Research

Monroe Berkowitz
Valerie Englander
Jeffrey Rubin
John D. Worrall

An Evaluation of Policy-Related Rehabilitation Research

PRAEGER SPECIAL STUDIES IN U.S. ECONOMIC, SOCIAL, AND POLITICAL ISSUES

Praeger Publishers   New York   Washington   London

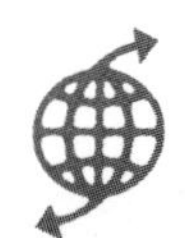

Library of Congress Cataloging in Publication Data
Main entry under title:

An Evaluation of policy-related rehabilitation
    research.

    (Praeger special studies in U. S. economic,
social, and political issues)
    Includes bibliographies and index.
    1. Rehabilitation research.   2. Rehabilitation.
I. Berkowitz, Monroe, 1919-
HD7255. E9   362. 8'5   75-23957
ISBN 0-275-01260-3

This book was prepared with the support of the National Science Foundation
Grant No. GI-39420. Any opinions, findings, conclusions, or recommendations
expressed are those of the author(s) and do not necessarily reflect the views of
the National Science Foundation.

PRAEGER PUBLISHERS
111 Fourth Avenue, New York, N.Y. 10003, U.S.A.

Published in the United States of America in 1975
by Praeger Publishers, Inc.

© 1975 by Bureau of Economic Research

Printed in the United States of America

This is a monograph about evaluation of research in the field of rehabilitation, written in 1974, at a time when the idea of "evaluation" has lost some of its glamor, promise, and hope. Much has changed since the Great Society's war to conquer poverty, cure urban ills, and usher in a better world was to be aided by rational calculation, whether in the form of program-planning-budgeting systems (PPBS), cost effectiveness, or systems analyses.

The manpower, training, and community-action programs are no longer expanding, and those that survived and those that have been abandoned seem distinguished more by political palatability than cost effectiveness. Through it all, the rehabilitation movement has grown and changed. The joint federal-state vocational-rehabilitation program played a part in many of the manpower programs, sometimes on a joint basis with the Office of Economic Opportunity and the Department of Labor. At a state level, some of the vocational-rehabilitation agencies combined in "umbrella" agencies with other manpower and social-service programs. Nationally, the Vocational Rehabilitation Agency, renamed the Rehabilitation Services Administration (RSA), became, for a time, part of a holding-company operation in the Social and Rehabilitation Service (SRS) within the Department of Health, Education, and Welfare.

But through it all, rehabilitation never lost its identity. Today, it is pulling back from some of its cooperative efforts, seeking to establish its role once again as the premier program to deal with the physically and mentally handicapped—and only peripherally with the culturally and socially disadvantaged.

In terms of dollars spent, rehabilitation programs are growing; rehabilitation research, too, although not growing at the pace desired by its administrators, shows a healthy stability. Our task in response to a National Science Foundation, Research Applied to National Needs (NSF, RANN) program proposal is to examine rehabilitation research and to evaluate its methodological quality and its policy utility.

The work is a multidisciplinary effort, but its editors are economists, who bring the biases of the profession to their task. Our training as economists insulated us from becoming too enthusiastic about the promise of evaluation and rational calculation in the administration of social programs in the 1960s. Unlike those administrators who viewed the principles of benefit-cost analysis as sacrosanct, we suspected that there were difficulties. We were under no illusion that

every valid theory and sound concept could be applied on a day-to-day
basis without consideration of institutional structures, political factors,
and human motivations. We recognized that some dimensions could
be measured easily, others only with difficulty, and that still others
would elude any measurement precise enough to be useful on a day-to-
day budgeting basis.

We have applied rational criteria to the evaluation of research
in the field of rehabilitation. At the same time, we recognize the wide
variety of motivations for doing research in this field. Some of the
studies we evaluated were research and demonstration projects that
were funded perhaps to provide services, to secure the cooperation
of professional groups, or to build a constituency for vocational
rehabilitation.

There was a time, perhaps 20 years ago, when any kind of
research in the field of rehabilitation was welcome. Merely arousing
the interest of any professional group in the field was a positive good
that could result in some program improvement. But now we know
that quality research can be done and that demonstration projects can
result in innovations. The time has come to take stock, to examine
the data, to investigate whether research can be improved, and to
inquire into the factors associated with quality research.

Certainly, a review and evaluation of the sort we undertake in
this book should not be interpreted as the final word on the research
program of any one agency or organization. Whatever its defects,
research has played an important role in the vast improvements seen
in the rehabilitation field in the past two decades. The dramatic
growth in the program is reviewed in Chapter 2. Our work should be
considered as another piece of information in a review of the quality
of research that has been carried out continuously by the rehabilitation agencies. The data generated by our project can serve as a
partial basis on which to build a framework for improvement in the
areas of research design and implementation and in the allocation of
research funds.

A number of agencies and individual researchers have provided
us with the final reports we reviewed in our undertaking. We are
grateful for their willingness to submit their work for review and
evaluation.

We recognize that many "scientific" precepts concerning sampling procedures, use of control groups, requirements for adequate
data base, and so on, are difficult to apply in this human-service
program. We further recognize that there will always be a need to
develop new areas (or perhaps new constituencies) to support the
program. But there is a continuing need to evaluate research as a
tool for seeking and applying knowledge. Therefore, we look at
rehabilitation research of many different types, processes, and

handicaps. In evaluating its methodology and policy utility, we make
recommendations aimed at improving quality standards in research.
Our belief is that better research can point the way to improved
rehabilitation programs.

This work would not have been started, had it not been for the
initiative of the NSF, RANN request for research proposals in this
area. It was supported by NSF, RANN 73-7 (Research Grant No.
GI-39420). Some of the problems we find with research in rehabilitation might well disappear if all grantees had the wise guidance and
direction we had from NSF, RANN personnel. We were never told
what to do or how to do it; our only requirement was to report on what
we did. Our reports were read intelligently and the suggestions we
received moved the project along in directions we thought useful and
sound. The responsibility for policy conclusions and remaining errors
and omissions rests with the researchers and, regrettably, cannot be
shared. The views expressed herein should not be ascribed as views
of the National Science Foundation.

This evaluation of policy-related research on rehabilitation is one of 20 in a series of projects on the Evaluation of Policy-Related Research in the Field of Human Resources, funded by the Division of Social Systems and Human Resources in the Research Applied to National Needs (RANN) program of the National Science Foundation.

A large body of policy-related research on human resources has been created over the past quarter-century. However, its usefulness to decision makers has been limited, because it has not been evaluated comprehensively with respect to technical quality, usefulness to policy makers, and potential for codification and wider diffusion. In addition, this research has been hard to locate and not easily accessible. Therefore, systematic and rigorous evaluations of this research are required to provide syntheses of evaluated information for use by public agencies at all levels of government and to aid in the planning and definition of research programs.

Recognizing those needs, the Division of Social Systems and Human Resources issued a Program Solicitation in January 1973 for proposals to evaluate policy-related research in 21 categories in the field of human resources. The competition resulted in 20 awards in June 1973. Each of the projects was to a) evaluate the internal validity of each study by determining whether the research used appropriate methods and data to deal with the questions asked; b) evaluate the external validity of the research by determining whether the results were credible in the light of other valid policy-related research; c) evaluate the policy utility of specific studies or sets of studies bearing on given policy instruments; d) provide decision makers, including research funders, with an assessed research base for alternative policy actions in a format readily interpretable and usable by decision makers. Each report was to include an analysis of the validity and utility of research in the field selected, a synthesis of the evidence, and a discussion of what, if any, additional research was required.

The following is a list of the awards, showing the research area evaluated, the organization to which the award was made, and the principal investigator:

1. An Evaluation of Policy-Related Research on New Expanded Roles of Health Workers. School of Medicine, Yale University, New Haven, Conn. 06520; Eva Cohen

2. An Evaluation of Policy-Related Research on the Effectiveness of
   Alternative Allocation of Health Care Manpower. Interstudy,
   123 East Grant Street, Minneapolis, Minn. 55403; Aaron Lowin
3. An Evaluation of Policy-Related Research on Effects of Health
   Care Regulation. Policy Center, Inc., Suite 500, 789 Sherman,
   Denver, Colo. 80203; Patrick O'Donoghue
4. An Evaluation of Policy-Related Research on Trade-offs Between
   Preventive and Primary Health Care. Boston University Medical
   Center, Boston University School of Medicine, Boston, Mass.
   02215; Paul Gertman
5. An Evaluation of Policy-Related Research on Effectiveness of
   Alternative Programs for the Handicapped. Rutgers University,
   165 College Avenue, New Brunswick, N.J. 08901; Monroe
   Berkowitz
6. An Evaluation of Policy-Related Research on Effects of Alterna-
   tive Health-Care-Reimbursement Systems. Department of
   Economics, University of Southern California, Los Angeles,
   Calif. 90007; Donald E. Yett
7. An Evaluation of Policy-Related Research on Alternative Public
   and Private Programs for Mid-life Redirection of Careers. Rand
   Corporation, 1700 Main Street, Santa Monica, Calif. 90406;
   Anthony H. Pascal
8. An Evaluation of Policy-Related Research on Relations Between
   Industrial Organization, Job Satisfaction, and Productivity.
   Florence G. Heller Graduate School for Advanced Studies in
   Social Welfare, Brandeis University, Waltham, Mass. 02154;
   Michael J. Brower
9. An Evaluation of Policy-Related Research on Relations Between
   Industrial Organization, Job Satisfaction, and Productivity.
   Department of Psychology, New York University, New York, N.Y.
   10003; Raymond A. Katzell
10. An Evaluation of Policy-Related Research on Productivity, Indus-
    trial Organization, and Job Satisfaction. School of Management,
    Case Western Reserve University, Cleveland, Ohio 44106;
    Suresh Srivastva
11. An Evaluation of Policy-Related Research on Effectiveness of
    Alternative Methods to Reduce Occupational Illness and Accidents.
    Westinghouse Behavioral Safety Center, Box 948, American City
    Building, Columbia, Md. 21044; Michael Pfeifer
12. An Evaluation of Policy-Related Research on the Impact of Union-
    ization on Public Institutions. Contract Research Corporation,
    25 Flanders Road, Belmont, Mass. 02178; Ralph Jones
13. An Evaluation of Policy-Related Research on Projection of Man-
    power Requirements. Center for Human Resources Research,
    Ohio State University, Columbus, Ohio 43210; S. C. Kelley

14. An Evaluation of Policy-Related Research on Effectiveness of
    Alternative Pretrial-Intervention Programs. ABT Associates,
    Inc., 55 Wheeler Street, Cambridge, Mass. 02138; Joan Mullen
15. An Evaluation of Policy-Related Research on Standards of Effec-
    tiveness for Pretrial-Release Programs. National Center for
    State Courts, 725 Madison Place, N.W., Washington, D.C. 20005;
    Barry Mahoney
16. An Evaluation of Policy-Related Research on Effectiveness of
    Volunteer Programs in the Area of Courts and Corrections.
    Department of Political Science, University of Illinois, Chicago
    Circle, Box 4348, Chicago, Ill. 60680; Thomas J. Cook
17. An Evaluation of Policy-Related Research on Effectiveness of
    Juvenile-Delinquency-Prevention Program. Department of
    Psychology, George Peabody College for Teachers, Nashville,
    Tenn. 37203; Michael C. Dixon
18. An Evaluation of Policy-Related Research on Exercise of Dis-
    cretion by Law-Enforcement Officials. College of William and
    Mary, Metropolitan Building, 147 Granby Street, Norfolk, Va.
    23510; W. Anthony Fitch
19. An Evaluation of Policy-Related Research on Exercise of Police
    Discretion. National Council of Crime and Delinquency Research
    Center, 609 Second Street, Davis, Calif. 95616; M. G. Neithercutt
20. An Evaluation of Policy-Related Research on Post Secondary
    Education for the Disadvantaged. Department of Sociology, Mercy
    College of Detroit, Detroit, Mich. 48219; Mary Janet Mulka

A complementary series of awards were made by the Division
of Social Systems and Human Resources to evaluate the policy-related
research in the field of Municipal Systems, Operations, and Services.
For the convenience of the reader, a listing of those awards appears
below:

1. Fire Protection. Department of Industrial and Systems Engineering, Georgia Institute of Technology, Atlanta, Ga. 30332;
   D. E. Fyffe
2. Fire Protection. New York Rand Institute, 545 Madison Avenue,
   New York, N.Y. 10022; Arthur J. Swersey
3. Emergency Medical Services. Bureau of Public Administration,
   University of Tennessee, Knoxville, Tenn. 37916; Hyrum Plaas
4. Municipal Housing Services. Cogen Holt and Associates, 956
   Chapel Street, New Haven, Conn. 06510; Harry Wexler
5. Formalized Pretrial Diversion Programs in Municipal and Metro-
   politan Courts. American Bar Association, 1705 DeSales Street,
   N.W., Washington, D.C. 20036; Roberta Rovner-Pieczenik

6. Parks and Recreation. National Recreation and Park Association, 1601 North Kent Street, Arlington, Va. 22209; The Urban Institute, 2100 M Street, N.W., Washington, D.C. 20037; Peter J. Verhoven

7. Police Protection. Mathematica, Inc., 4905 Del Ray Avenue, Bethesda, Md. 20014; Saul I. Gass

8. Solid-Waste Management. Department of Engineering, Massachusetts Institute of Technology, Cambridge, Mass. 02139; David Marks

9. Citizen Participation Strategies. The Rand Corporation, 2100 M Street, N.W., Washington, D.C. 20037; Robert Yin

10. Citizen Participation: Municipal Subsystems. Program in Health Planning, The University of Michigan, Ann Arbor, Mich. 48104; Joseph L. Falkson

11. Economic Development. Ernst & Ernst, 1225 Connecticut Avenue, N.W., Washington, D.C. 20036; Lawrence H. Revzan

12. Goal of Economic Development. Center for Economic Development, Department of Economics, University of Texas, Austin, Austin, Tex. 78712; Niles M. Hansen

13. Franchising and Regulation. Department of Economics, University of South Dakota, Vermillion, S.D. 57069; C. A. Kent

14. Municipal-Information Systems. Public Policy Research Organization, University of California, Irvine, Irvine, Calif. 92664; Kenneth L. Kraemer

15. Municipal-Growth Guidance Systems. School of Public Affairs, University of Minnesota, Minneapolis, Minn. 55455; Michael E. Gleeson

16. Land-Use Controls. Center for Urban and Regional Studies, University of North Carolina, Chapel Hill, Chapel Hill, N. Car. 27514; Edward M. Bergman

17. Land-Use Controls. The Potomac Institute, Inc., 1501 Eighteenth Street, N.W., Washington, D.C. 20036; Herbert M. Franklin

18. Municipal Management Methods and Budgetary Processes. The Urban Institute, 2100 M Street, N.W., Washington, D.C. 20037; Wayne A. Kimmel

19. Personnel Systems. Georgetown University, Public Service Laboratory, Washington, D.C. 20037; Selma Mushkin

Copies of the research evaluation reports for both Municipal Systems and Human Resources cited above may be obtained directly from the principal investigators or from the National Technical Information Service (NTIS), U.S. Dept. of Commerce, 5285 Port Royal, Springfield, Va. 22151; telephone (703) 321-8517.

This research evaluation by Monroe Berkowitz of the Disability and Health Economics Research Section of the Bureau of Economic

Research of Rutgers University on the effectiveness of alternative
programs for the handicapped was prepared with the support of the
National Science Foundation. The opinions, findings, conclusions, or
recommendations are solely those of the authors.

It is a policy of the Division of Social Systems and Human
Resources to assess the relevance, utility, and quality of the projects
it supports. Should any readers of this book have comments in those
or other regards, we would be particularly grateful to receive them,
as they become essential tools in the planning of future programs.

Lynn P. Dolins
Program Manager
Division of Social Systems
and Human Resources

This work evaluates the methodological adequacy and policy utility of research in the area of rehabilitation of the handicapped. The analysis was based on a multidisciplinary review of a sample (477) of project reports chosen from more than 4,000 reports screened. A summarized version of each report was obtained by having a checklist completed by a student in the field. The resulting summary, along with the actual final report, was forwarded to a faculty member who rated the report on its methodological adequacy and policy utility.

Each of the individual panel members contributed a chapter reviewing a group of reports related to a specific field: social work, behavior modification, psychiatric rehabilitation, public offenders, special education, vocational education, adolescents, and organizational matters in rehabilitation. Also, separate chapters deal with correlates of success and benefit-cost studies.

In general, we found a poor level of methodology in most of the research that in turn helped to keep the policy-utility ratings low (although the rating distribution on the policy aspect of research was above that of methodology). Tabular presentations indicate that NIMH as a grantor did better than others. Universities and university medical schools were the best grantees in our sample. Surprisingly, state vocational rehabilitation agencies did poorly in policy utility (a result conditioned by the poor methodology found in many of their studies).

Other variables identified as significant in our regression analysis were statistical analysis (positively affected success criteria), sampling that entered doubt about program generalizability (negative effect), evaluation by people involved in the program (negative effect on methodology only), and a clear statement of hypothesis (positive effect).

The results of our overall analysis, as well as that provided by the individual panel members, led to suggestions designed to improve the research-grant structure. The most significant of the resulting recommendations were as follows: the clear statement of objectives of the research program; postproject review; the building of a constituency that would demand quality research; the separation of the service aspects of a program from its research and evaluation component; and the attainment of a better relationship between practitioners and researchers to assure that appropriate research topics are designed and that the results have policy utility.

CONTENTS

THE PROBLEM, ITS SETTING, AND OUR APPROACH

The research for this work originated with a National Science Foundation grant to the Bureau of Economic Research at Rutgers University. As part of its Research Applied to National Needs (RANN) series, NSF sought research proposals designed to evaluate the effectiveness of alternative programs for the handicapped. Our assignment was formidable; we were faced with a plethora of options. Our first step was to limit the project to the field of rehabilitation, and then to review rehabilitation research to specify and delimit the material to be analyzed. Such a review would provide some measure of the effectiveness of a number of programs in providing training, counseling, and other services to the handicapped and disabled. In our efforts to define the scope and range of our project, we had to answer the following questions: What should we consider rehabilitation research? How does one go about identifying and locating that research? From what analytical perspective can the most useful results be attained?

The proposal by the Bureau of Economic Research, therefore, focused on rehabilitation research, with special emphasis on design and methodology. Since the field of rehabilitation research and the handicapped covers a number of academic disciplines, we suggested that a panel of experts in a variety of rehabilitation-related areas be chosen to aid in the evaluation. We anticipated that those panel members would contribute chapters that would relate the literature in their fields to the work done by practitioners as well as to their general discipline.

Before embarking upon a detailed discussion of the mechanics of this project, we shall attempt a more precise delineation of the nature of our study.

THE LIMITS OF OUR INQUIRY

Our primary goal was to determine and assess the contributions to rehabilitation practice that have been made by a number of research programs and projects. Specifically, we sought data on the approaches that worked in particular situations and on the kind of disabled individuals with which they worked. The approaches varied from technical procedures to hospital treatments to organizational restructuring, and so on. The object of our analysis was to determine whether some consistency and agreement existed as to the effectiveness of alternative treatments so that practitioners would have a better notion of the direction in which they should go and of their prospects for success. Our hope was to help save time, money, and perhaps lives in the end.

Our secondary objective was to help improve the quality of research in the field of rehabilitation. That was attempted in two ways: by highlighting the pitfalls encountered by past researchers and by identifying the methodological aspects of successful research efforts.

SOURCES OF RESEARCH REPORTS

Our first task in attempting to achieve our stated objectives was to identify the relevant research. Our original reliance on abstracts culled from contacting rehabilitation and service agencies resulted in data that were not only insufficient but were frequently duplicative as well. We therefore decided to limit our search to the two major sources of abstracts on rehabilitation research: the Social and Rehabilitation Service (SRS) of HEW and the Smithsonian Science Information Exchange (SSIE). The SRS had previously abstracted all of the final reports on the projects they had funded between 1954 and 1972, and the SSIE had available abstracts on projects funded by a variety of governmental and private agencies from 1954 through 1973. It was felt that those two agencies would provide us with as representative and as broad a spectrum of research in rehabilitation as we would have been able to obtain through our contacts with 140 rehabilitation-related public and private agencies and library services.

Although we had thought that the abstracts alone would provide enough information for our purposes, we soon discovered that they were not adequate. We therefore decided to obtain copies of the complete final reports of those projects that met our screening criteria.

SCREENING CRITERIA

To allocate the limited resources we had it was necessary to
limit the size of the sample of reports we would review. We developed
a set of screening criteria with the intent of including only those reports that contained a description and evaluation of a program of
rehabilitation, which we defined as the alteration of a disabling char-
acteristic or its consequences. A standard of that type meant that we
would examine a wide spectrum of research including reports of the
so-called "research and demonstration" (R&D) projects. Demonstrations without any discernible research component—e.g., descriptions
of service activities or attempts to install a proven program in a
familiar setting—were not included. On the other hand, R&D projects
that sought to test a relationship between variables or to test a program
in a more general setting and that reported the results of the research
or evaluation were admitted to our sample. Some would argue that
holding R&D projects to tests based on the scientific requirements of
research is unfair. However, a significant portion of rehabilitation
research funds are directed to those projects. Whatever the motivation for the funding or the carrying out of the activities, those projects
report results that purport to have general applicability. Such results
presumably are meant to be applied elsewhere; they represent the
findings derived from the experiment and from the demonstration. If
the results are to be credible and valid, they must meet the kind of
design, analysis, and utility criteria our checklist was meant to
examine.

On the basis of our screening criteria we eliminated all reports
that lacked a research or evaluation component for a rehabilitation
program. Reports in a number of general categories fell out of our
sample on that basis. Those included service programs, case studies
involving fewer than 15 participants, surveys that did not include a
correlates-of-success component, teaching guides or manuals, planning studies, and architectural barrier studies. Even with those kinds
of reports eliminated, we were left with a sample much too large for
comprehensive individual analysis. Therefore, we also chose to
exclude medical and surgical research; studies whose primary concentration was testing, tool development, and evaluation; bioengineering, mobility, and orientation studies; and studies of attitudes of
nonrehabilitants.

We felt that those involved in the medical aspects of rehabilitation
would benefit little from a review of their research—medical journals
and other sources undoubtedly already provide adequate and up-to-
date information. Furthermore, a cursory review of some of the

medical projects we received revealed that they were distinctly different (i.e., design oriented) from the majority of rehabilitation research. There is no doubt that such an exclusion creates a bias in our sample. Given the existence of such a bias, the reader should be cautious in attempting to generalize our conclusions to all rehabilitation research and especially to the kinds of projects we screened out. * The best generalizations would likely be those made in light of the special nature of our sample.

Similar reasoning was applied in eliminating of tool-development and bioengineering studies. And as for testing, we selected only those reports in which tests were applied in a rehabilitation program. For example, a report detailing differences between retardates and normals in a test series, while perhaps providing useful information, could not be said to have immediate implications for finding out what works in the process of rehabilitation. It was on that process of rehabilitation, entailing intake, plan of services, and outcome, that we focused. If a report failed to be specifically oriented toward one or more steps in this process, we chose to eliminate it.

Despite our rigorous screening process, we allowed for two special cases: correlates-of-success or outcome studies and cost-benefit studies, the first for their overall significance and the second for their special relationship to the authors' own orientation. Outcome studies, although not meeting our formal criteria (they are more statistical than program oriented), were included because of their bearing on our overall goal; they afford a statistical determination of the significant variables related to success in rehabilitation programs. Such research offers the promise of providing standards for policy makers for the recruitment and selection of clients for programs. In regard to the second special case, that of the cost-benefit studies of rehabilitation programs, we discuss their rationale, usefulness, limitations, and implications when applied to rehabilitation research.

EVALUATIVE METHOD EMPLOYED

Once we had screened all the abstracts provided by SRS and SSIE, we then had to obtain copies of all the final reports we had chosen to include in our research. Our next task was to develop a special checklist (see Appendix A), designed for two purposes: to gather relevant data for an overall analysis and to provide relevant

---

* Generalizing past the years 1955-73 may be dangerous, also, if major changes in the conduct of research occurred after that time.

information for panel members.[*] The latter were drawn largely from faculty in appropriate rehabilitation-related fields. Their assignment was to rate the research on its methodological adequacy and policy utility, as well as to evaluate its external validity.

For the checklisting of the reports, we hired graduate students in the appropriate rehabilitation-related fields, and, when necessary, undergraduates with majors in the relevant fields of inquiry were also used. To assure consistent answers to our checklist questions, we prepared a detailed instruction sheet and held orientation sessions on the use of the checklist. We also had the panel members choose a graduate student with whom they were familiar to work as a funnel through which reports could be siphoned for review. When the panel member finished with a report, his findings were coded and the information was then keypunched. An overall analysis of the data appears in Chapter 14.

The Checklist

Project Background and Particulars

The first two pages of the checklist sought general information about the author, grantee, grantor, academic discipline, and handicap. A description of the project in general terms and by the stages of the rehabilitation process was included, as were the length of the report and the duration and funding of the project. Unfortunately, our information on funding tended to be incomplete. For most SRS projects we have the amount of funds provided by SRS, but our figures do not

---

[*]The numbers associated with this process are total number of abstracts received (4,146); screened out on first review (2,064); and requested for further review (2,082) reports. On receipt of more information 1,008 were rejected. We were unable to get 597 reports for some of the following reasons: the project was continuing; it was actually a service program; no final report was written; and so on. Many of our postcards, letters, and follow-up letters went unanswered; in other cases, reports were received at such a late date that their inclusion was impossible (a number of microfiche reports were in this category, due to an administrative mix-up). Had we received those reports, there is no question that many would have been screened out on further examination. In all we ended with 477 reports to be checklisted and rated. Based on a comparison of the abstracts of the reports not received with the reports received, we feel the 477 reports adequately represent the field we sought to examine.

necessarily represent the total funding. Funding data for non-SRS projects were even sketchier: funding for Veterans Administration (VA) projects was unavailable; funding for National Institutes of Health (NIH) projects was available but subject to the same limitations as found in SRS. It was also impossible to obtain adequate data on the funding of projects supported by state government or private agencies and foundations.

<u>Sampling</u>

The second section of the checklist pertained to the sampling used in the research. Included was a description of the sample, its selection, and its size. The reviewer was then asked to comment on the generalizability of the results, given the researchers' sampling techniques. Two important and related questions are raised in that section. First, if the researchers used a sample, was it a true representation of the population under discussion? The second question concerns the use of a screening mechanism for "research clients": were clients selected by a choice process that affected the likelihood of project success?

In regard to the first question, the answers on the checklist indicate that a true sample was not chosen in the majority of cases. It was of prime importance that the researcher not seek to generalize past his limited population. It is best to remember that without a valid sampling technique, the results are limited in applicability to people with characteristics similar to those of the people involved in the study. The determination of the personal, demographic, social, and physical characteristics that are relevant is no easy matter. Even for people with the same handicap, the significant characteristics may differ, depending on the type and/or method of rehabilitation pursued. For that reason a more detailed identification, either through the use of a control group or by statistical methods, is essential.

The second question, concerning screening procedures, is most assuredly an important one. For although a research project may continually prove successful, its applicability may be limited due to its concentration on clients with the greatest rehabilitation potential. It should be noted, however, that screening does not invalidate the results but only limits their applicability. The extent to which the limitation occurs depends not only on the strictness of the screening but also on the size of the disabled population treated during the research project: The larger the population, the more generalizations one can make about the probable future benefits from wide-scale introduction of the technique tested in the project. The implications for benefit-cost review of research projects will be examined in Chapter 13.

Data Gathering

In the third section of the checklist, information was sought on
sources of data and techniques for gathering facts. The reviewer noted
whether subjective or objective client ratings were used, who made
those ratings, and what kinds of tests were given to the clients. We
also wanted to know about the existence and treatment of nonresponses,
refusals, and/or dropouts. Unfortunately, due to the way the question
was phrased and to the lack of information in most of the reports, the
checklist was unable to provide great detail here.

Project Design and Follow-up

The fourth section of the checklist included an examination of
the experimental design of the project (see Campbell and Stanley,
1966), data on the use of control groups, randomization, and nonexperimental techniques. That information provided the panel member with
a quick view of the experimental set-up and allowed us to examine the
effect of design on policy utility and methodology. Parenthetically,
the most often used design was the one-shot case study. The use of
the generally accepted "better" designs, such as the pretest/posttest
control group and the posttest-only control group was found to be
limited. The former was found 42 times (8.8 percent), and the latter
was used 28 times (5.9 percent).

A project's experimental design is an important consideration
in assessing the results of the research and hence should be of great
concern to those involved in rehabilitation. If the design lacks strong
controls, the results may be thrown open to question, thereby delaying
the implementation of what could be a useful and effective program.

We next explored differential methods of client follow-up. By
"follow-up" we meant a review of client status at some stage after the
original project had terminated. Since the assumption is that during
the period from the conclusion of the project to the follow-up, the
clients were left to their own devices, any comparisons between the
control and experimental groups would indicate the true impact of the
project and not of the project plus some further services. Critical to
this definition is the nontreatment of program participants in the period
between the conclusion of the project and the follow-up survey.

Treatment and Outcome Variables

Our next concern was with determining the research variables—
specifically, the treatment provided and the outcome it produced. The
data on treatment variables provide some notion of the practical application of particular combinations of intake methods and services.

TABLE 1.1

Treatment Variables

Treatment	Number of Times Used[*]
Counseling	178
Vocational training	177
Placement services	105
Evaluation (vocational)	78
Sheltered workshop	56
Psychiatric help	47
Medical treatment	39
Physical therapy	38
Social work	37
Special education	33
Evaluation (medical)	31
On-the-job training	27
Halfway house	21
Speech therapy	13
Team counseling	11
Attitude changes	10
Outreach interviews	8
Income maintenance	6
School	5
Hospital care (inpatient)	5
Hospital care (outpatient)	3
Information publicity	3

[*]This includes the number of times the treatment was the sole aspect of the program, as well as the times it was used in concert with other treatments. The reader should be aware that the numbers are inexact, since they come from coded information in response to a general question on the checklist. To keep the number of codes down to manageable proportions, the coder was asked to fit the described treatment into one of 97 possible combinations; hence, some minor aspects of the treatment programs may have been lost.

When the outcome measures are brought into the picture some idea of
the rehabilitation process as a whole will emerge. That, in turn, leads
to an understanding of the effectiveness of the alternatives open to the
practitioner.

Table 1.1 indicates the frequency with which various kinds of
treatment were provided in our sample. The treatments include services, facilities, tests, and other forms of assistance, as well as the
locations in which they might be administered. Most striking in
Table 1.1 is the relatively high frequency of traditional rehabilitation
methods—i.e., counseling and job-related activities. The pattern con-
firms the representativeness of our sample. The four most-used
combinations were a) counseling, vocational training, and placement
services; b) counseling, vocational evaluation, and vocational training;
c) vocational evaluation, vocational training, and placement services,
and d) counseling, vocational training, and a sheltered workshop.

The most frequent outcome variable was employment (168 times).
A simple success/failure or rehabilitated/not rehabilitated designation
for outcomes was found a number of times: 98 and 50 times, respec-
tively. The five next most significant outcomes were recidivism* (45
times), change in functioning capacity (41 times), change in client
attitude (37 times), and the attainment of an independent living style
and a change in self-concept (both 35 times). Those outcomes offer
no surprises and help to reconfirm our sampling procedures.

Client Characteristics

In the next portion of our checklist we tried to provide our
reviewers with some information as to the controls that were found
in the project report. We used a four-part question for each of a
number of demographic, disability and socioeconomic variables. For
each variable we wanted to know whether it was considered, analyzed
or described, or controlled, and if the last, whether that control was
weak or strong. A variable was to be marked "considered" if it was
mentioned at all in the report. In essence, that meant that the
researcher was aware of the importance of the variable but was unable
or chose not to look into it further. A check in the category "effects
analyzed or described" indicated that an after-the-fact analysis of
the impact on outcome of a particular variable had been undertaken.
Such an analysis usually involved an attempt to locate any significant
differences between groups by the use of a t or chi-square statistical
test.

---

*Recidivism could mean either a return to prison or a hospital.

In determining the presence and strength of controls, the distinction between weak and strong control was not always clear. The former generally meant an imperfectly matched control group, while the latter indicated either that both control groups and experimental groups were randomly assigned or that a statistical technique, such as multiple regression analysis, was employed. In some cases, strong control existed as a result of the limited nature of the particular client group— i.e., the disability of each client might have been the same, the clients might have been drawn from one age group, and so on. The variables most often controlled were age, sex, and disability; those least controlled were prior military status, ethnicity, and religion. As for the importance of controlling specific variables, the reader should review Chapter 11 on correlates of success; it examines the many findings of previous studies on the variables most often related to outcome in rehabilitation programs, providing the reader with the information needed to draw conclusions about the controls found in the reports in our sample. An examination of the impact of controls on methodology rating can be found in Chapter 14.

Statistical and Analytical Techniques

The next section of the checklist concerned the use of associational, correlation, and/or multivariate analysis. It was included in order to give the panel members and our readers some idea of the statistical sophistication of recent rehabilitation research. The extent to which each of those methods was found in our sample can be seen in Table 1.2. As expected, the more sophisticated techniques were used least often. (The impact of statistical analysis on methodological rating is also examined in Chapter 14.)

TABLE 1.2

Statistical Analyses Used

	Yes	No	No Response or Not Applicable	Total
Associational analysis	168	271	38	477
	(35.29)	(56.90)	(10.19)	(100)
Correlation analysis	81	365	31	477
	(16.99)	(76.50)	(6.59)	(100)
Multivariate analysis	58	375	44	477
	(12.29)	(78.69)	(9.29)	(100)

Note: Numbers in parentheses are percentages.

<u>Validity and Implications for Implementation</u>

The final section of the checklist provided a review of the validity and the policy utility of a particular report. Among the questions it raised were the following: Does the research contradict existing knowledge? Is it possible to implement the kinds of programs suggested by the research? How amenable to manipulation are the independent variables, and will their manipulation significantly affect the outcome? After he can considered those and similar questions, the panel member was asked to rate the overall project on its methodology and policy utility. Each of the separate rating scales used was a simple 1 (low) to 10 (high). Unfortunately, little significance can be attached to those data, for a variety of reasons. Since the panel members have widely divergent academic backgrounds, their attitudes toward methodology and policy utility are notably disparate. For example, some of our raters specialized in methodology and research design, while others were more concerned with applicability and significance for real-world problems. In other words, if two panel members read the same report they might rationally come up with varying scores. Another factor affecting ratings is a definitional one, stemming from individual variations in intuitive definitions of words such as "good" and "high." A final reason for the noncongruence of the ratings is traceable to the assignment of reports to panel members based on their discipline. And there is the possibility of qualitative differences among groups of reports. It is these differences that we were trying to isolate. To identify possible biases arising from such specialization, we had all the panel members evaluate a subgroup of seven reports. It was thus possible to test for significant differences between raters. Through an analysis of variance test we identified two groups of raters for policy utility and for methodology. Within each group no significant difference existed in their ratings for our test sample of reports.

Some Possible Biases—Ours and Theirs

Having concluded our discussion of the checklist, we think it might prove useful to examine some of the shortcomings of the instrument that have come to light since our study began. First, we found that the nature of the checklist tended to make our panel members overly critical, emphasizing departures from scientific research. Second, much of the impact of a piece of research was ignored, since we were forced to view one project at a time and considered none in its overall context in a research plan. A third difficulty was the previously mentioned lack of consistency among checklisters.

Additional bias undoubtedly existed due to the nature of our screening criteria. Although quality was not a factor in screening, other aspects of the sorting process might have affected our final sample. For example, should the nature of the research universe be such that SRS and SSIE are not representative, our conclusions would obviously lack the generalizability we were seeking. One area in which our sample is weak is that of unsupported research done at universities and hospitals and later published in journals, a type that may represent the most scientific research, since journals generally impose strict requirements on the material they publish. However, that bias is counteracted to some extent by the existence of poor projects that are never concluded and hence go unreported.

Another bias results from our exclusive focus on material presented in a final-report format. We therefore had to bypass those funded projects that did not require a formal report. In other instances we were forced to rely on a short summary or some other published or unpublished material made available to us.

THE IMPACT OF ALTERNATIVE MOTIVATIONS
UPON EVALUATION

We have assumed that most research has been conducted in order to expand knowledge about rehabilitation, either through basic, first-hand inquiry or through the application of existing knowledge to experimental situations. Most of the projects we reviewed fell into the latter category, testing existing ideas about the provision of services in new environments or on different clients. We may have missed a good deal of basic research by our decision to screen out medical rehabilitation research. But since our chief concern was to evaluate rehabilitative techniques, we chose to concentrate upon research that modified existing practices and knowledge. In so doing, we mean to impute no less significance to basic research, for it is the seed of existing knowledge.

Another possible justification for rehabilitation research is the need to build a constituency of supporters. The funders may therefore be less concerned with the particulars of the research than they are with involving special types of researchers in the study of rehabilitation. Similarly, funds ostensibly for research might be used to buy support for the general idea of rehabilitation from a particular set of persons. In either case, the resulting evaluation might well miss the point.

One must keep in mind that the goals of both the grantee and the grantor may diverge from methodological purity and policy utility.

For example, given a set of research proposals, some of which are in different areas, a funder, having examined the goals and objectives of the grantees, may decide to fund a project based on considerations other than the likely validity of the experimental design. One set of proposals may involve an area that has been thoroughly reviewed and researched and where design consequently poses little problem, whereas another set may involve an approach to rehabilitation that has never been examined. The funder's selection of the latter may result in a lower methodological quality, but the final study may well have more overall usefulness.

The researcher's motivation also affects what gets done and how. His research may be affected by such considerations as his practical and academic background, his desire to benefit other members of society, and his individual talents and interests. He may be motivated by enhanced academic prestige, opportunities for promotion, the building of a research section, and even the desire to make a profit. On a different level, some practitioners may need to prove the effectiveness of their own efforts. None of these motives for doing research can be faulted unless it interferes with an unbiased, reasoned, and relevant research project.

THE DEVELOPMENT OF AN EVALUATION PERSPECTIVE

Recent years have seen a rapid expansion in the area of evaluation (Niskanen, 1973; Weiss, 1972; Rivlin, 1971; Wholey, 1970). A number of different historical trends have contributed to the kind of evaluation currently being done. Those trends come out of academic disciplines, government regulations, and the social and the political environment, among others.

The academic discipline that has had perhaps the most to do with the tools of evaluation has been economics. In the past decades cost-benefit analysis, a long-established but little used tool, has come to the forefront in the work of many applied economists. Its popularity reflects the increasing general concern with public spending in a time of rapidly growing government expenditures at all levels. Presumably, cost-benefit analysis serves as a guide for an efficient allocation of funds. The refinement and enhanced availability of that tool has provided researchers and decision makers with some gauge of the effectiveness of various programs, among them the whole area of rehabilitation.

A second academic discipline that has contributed to evaluation is the field of research or experimental design. Perhaps the work of Campbell and Stanley best epitomizes the efforts in this area. They discuss in great detail the need for, uses of, and pitfalls in various experimental designs. That widely accepted work provides researchers with a theoretical and practical framework for conducting quality research.

Forces outside academia have also affected evaluative procedures (Rossi and Williams, 1972, pp. 11-49). The rapid expansion of government social welfare programs in the 1960s is one such force. Many of those programs had vague although generally acceptable goals. Unlike the New Deal programs, whose value could be shown by the simplicity and the immediacy of their goals (such as employment), more recent expenditures have not specified short-term, meaningful, and measurable outcomes. Their eventual failure and collapse prompted the federal government to seek ways to determine the programs that were working, as well as the ways for, the reasons for, and the extent of their success. Legislation began, therefore, to require that evaluation be an integral part of various social-welfare projects. Funds were thus available for social scientists to conduct research and evaluations. Such federal funding no doubt attracted many scholars to what had once been considered the uninteresting fields of methodology and evaluation.

Examples of the outcome of the process can be found in recent research projects sponsored by the SRS. One of the most extensive of those projects was undertaken by Collignon and associates at the Institute of Urban and Regional Development of the University of California at Berkeley. Their work has resulted in surveys of evaluation procedures, outlines for cost-benefit analysis, and historical reviews of work in the rehabilitation field.

Another SRS grant resulted in the development of the Analytic Aids for Research Proposal Selection (AARPS) at the Texas Institute for Rehabilitation and Research. That program (discussed in Chapter 13) was designed to establish a cost-benefit review of research proposals so that research funds could be allocated more efficiently. And another project (discussed in greater detail in Chapter 14) is currently being undertaken by John Muthard and staff at the Regional Rehabilitation Research Institute of the University of Florida. Their major thrust is upon measuring the impact of several selected R&D projects and the consideration of that impact in relation to the quality of the research. They are especially interested in determining whether research has to meet minimum requirements before it can have some effect on what is practiced in the field.

Still another project currently underway is that of Willy De Geyndt at Minnesota Systems Research Inc., who is analyzing the methodological adequacy of a selected set of SRS-funded projects. His investigation covers several aspects of research design (sampling, statistics, and objectives), as well as the factors relating to the quality of the methodology.

In general, then, we can see that the trends toward research evaluation, more efficient allocation of expenditures, and improved research tools have jointly resulted in disparate projects whose shared aim is to determine the effectiveness of funded R&D projects. When completed, those projects will provide a fuller picture of the history, quality, impact, and overall effectiveness of a large part of rehabilitation research.

PLAN OF REPORT

The next chapter reviews the federal-state rehabilitation program. Chapter 3 discusses the historical development and current status of rehabilitation research. It will be followed by a group of chapters from our panel members in which they review the research they examined and offer recommendations concerning rehabilitation policy and research procedure. The remaining chapters view the overall data from our project and attempt to determine whether any conclusions can be reached about the relationship between methodological quality, policy utility, and some of the significant checklist variables. A final section details our findings and their implications for funders, researchers, practitioners, and the disabled.

REFERENCES

Campbell, D. T., and Stanley, J. C. _Experimental and Quasi-Experimental Designs for Research_. Chicago: Rand McNally, 1966.

Niskanen, W. A. _Benefit-Cost and Policy Analysis—1972_. Chicago: Aldine, 1973.

Rivlin, A. M. _Systematic Thinking for Social Action_. Washington, D.C.: The Brookings Institution, 1971.

Rossi, P. H., and Williams, W., eds. _Evaluating Social Programs: Theory, Practice and Politics_. New York: Seminar Press, 1972.

Weiss, C. _Evaluation Research: Methods of Assessing Program Effectiveness_. Englewood Cliffs, N.J.: Prentice-Hall, 1972.

Wholey, J. S. _Federal Evaluation Policy: Analyzing the Effects of Public Programs_. Washington, D.C.: The Urban Institute, 1970.

More than a million persons (1,176,445) were served by the
state vocational rehabilitation agencies in 1973.[*] About 30 percent
of that number (360,726) were successfully rehabilitated.[†] Each
state agency operates under a federal grant-in-aid program, with the
federal government providing 80 percent of the funds and the remaining 20 percent coming from matching state funds.

We have almost no comprehensive data on rehabilitation activity
in the private sector and only sketchy data on the rehabilitation activities in other public agencies. There is reason to believe, however,
that state vocational rehabilitation agencies provided or arranged for
services for about one-fifth of the total cases in 1966 (Treitel, 1970,
Table 5, p. 20). If this proportion has held constant, the likelihood
is that five million persons had some contact with rehabilitation
programs in 1973.

---

[*]Each state, as well as Washington, D.C., Guam, Puerto Rico,
and the Virgin Islands, has a general vocational rehabilitation agency
that serves clients with all physical and mental disabilities. In addition, 28 states have specialized agencies for the blind. In recent
years, several of the agencies have amalgamated together with other
social service offices in an umbrella-type agency within the state.

[†]This is referred to as "closure 26," which indicates that a
client is placed in gainful employment or homemaking activity upon
completion of a plan of services jointly devised by the client and the
rehabilitation counselor.

ILLNESS AND DISABILITIES

Definitional confusion is manifest in the rehabilitation field. In order to clarify our usage of certain terms, we should review and identify the various stages of the disability process. The process begins with an injury or disease, perhaps a traumatic insult or the invasion of a body by a virus. The injury or disease may result in an impairment, which is a physical or mental abnormality, perhaps the reduction of heart or lung capacity, loss of muscle tone, deleterious change in blood pressure, and so on. The impairment may lead to a functional limitation, such as difficulty in seeing, hearing, lifting, stooping, walking, and so forth, and the functional limitation may lead in turn to a disability, which is defined as a change in the person's role functioning. In the case of most male adults between the ages of 18 and 64 disability is defined in terms of their inability to participate in the labor force or in other work activities.

While it is helpful to visualize the disability process as a chain, we do not wish to imply that long periods of time must pass between stages or that a person need experience each stage. A person who suffers injury that results in impairment and that leads to a functional limitation does not necessarily become "disabled," as we have defined it. Perhaps the function that is limited is not essential to the job; perhaps the employer can alter work requirements, or sheer determination on the part of the injured person may overcome the limitation. On the other hand, a mild functional limitation—say, restriction of movement of the arms—can be disastrous to a laborer whose limited education, geographic location, or family circumstances preclude alternative employment.

RESTORING THE DISABLED

After World War I, in 1921, the rehabilitation movement began in an organized fashion in the public sector. It was designed to help the injured person or the chronically ill to avert the disability status. Its overwhelming emphasis was on orthopedic disability. Rehabilitationists are fond of defining rehabilitation as the process of restoring the handicapped to the fullest mental, physical, social, and vocational levels of which they are capable. The distinguishing hallmark of rehabilitation was that it could utilize a variety of services to accomplish the desired objective.

When the movement began to develop in the United States, the rehabilitation agencies were usually located in the vocational education

department of the state government, and, consequently, vocational
training was stressed. However, other services were introduced over
time. Since 1943 the state agencies have had the authority to spend
funds for medical restoration of a person once preliminary medical
care has stabilized his physical condition.

Clients must first of all be admitted to the rehabilitation program
in the individual state. Who should or should not be admitted is dependent upon the discretion exercised by state agencies. The discretion
is bounded by the requirement that eligibility be based on the presence
of a disability that creates a substantial handicap to employment, with
a reasonable expectation that vocational rehabilitation (VR) services
will result in rehabilitation. In recent years client groups have been
playing a role in such decisions, but admittance is not a right that is
enforceable by law.

Once admitted, a client may be given physical restoration and
therapy services designed to minimize impairment or, if the impairment exists, to avert functional limitation. If there is a residual
limitation, the client may be offered training in an educational program designed to minimize disability. All services provided are in
accordance with an individual plan of services worked out with the
counselor and tailored to the individual client's needs. The counselor
in charge of the case may provide counseling, guidance, and eventually
aid in placing the person in a job. Most of the services provided, be
they training, education, physical restoration, physical therapy, or
testing, will be purchased. Although partially dependent on public
funds, the services are provided by the private sector. We should
also reiterate that a good deal of vocational rehabilitation is handled
in the private sector and in other public agencies.

The Veterans Administration (VA) has its own rehabilitation
program, and we shall examine later some of the research that it con-
ducts and some that it funds. Since rehabilitation activity is intimately
connected with medical programs, the various parts of the Public Health
Service, particularly the National Institutes of Health (NIH) and the
National Institutes of Mental Health (NIMH), are concerned with
rehabilitation. For the most part, those agencies fund rehabilitation
research but do not directly provide rehabilitation services. General
and specialized hospitals, medical schools, and other institutes are
providers of some rehabilitation services, and they conduct training
programs and rehabilitation research. It is useful for purposes of
trends to look at the joint federal-state programs, but we must always
be conscious of the fact that we are only looking at a portion of rehabilitation activity in the country.

GROWTH IN THE FEDERAL-STATE
REHABILITATION PROGRAM

By almost any measure—the number of people served, the number of people rehabilitated, or the amount of expenditures—the state rehabilitation program has grown steadily over the years. In 1921, 500 persons were rehabilitated. In 1938, when data on the number of persons served were first collected in a systematic fashion, nearly 64,000 cases were served. Five years later, at the beginning of the war period, the number was more than 100,000 a year. At the conclusion of the war, the number again doubled. The half million mark was reached in the mid-1960s, and the decade of the 1970s began with more than 1 million cases being served each year. The numbers have more than kept pace with changes in population: In 1963, fewer than 200 persons per 100,000 population were being served; the number had swelled to 557 per 100,000 population by 1973.

The state program relies not so much on the number of cases served as on the number of persons "rehabilitated" as an indicator of success. In the evaluation of our research projects, however, we will rate several measures of outcome in addition to "rehabilitated" or "not rehabilitated." Suffice it to say, for purposes of classification, a rehabilitant is defined as a person who is placed in a job (or, in the case of a homemaker, restored to functioning in homemaking activities) and remains in that status for a period of 60 days or more. (Until recently, 30 days had been the required time, although local practice in some offices allowed for 60 days for the severely disabled.)

As shown in Table 2.1, during the 1930s the number of rehabilitants averaged about 10,000 each year. World War II saw the numbers double and then quadruple. Shortly after the war, 50,000 persons each year were being rehabilitated. The program significantly expanded in the 1950s and growth has continued until the present day, when more than 300,000 persons are rehabilitated each year. In terms of the proportion of population, again, the rate of rehabilitation has increased considerably. In 1963, 58 persons per 100,000 population in the United States were being rehabilitated; by 1973, 171 out of 100,000 achieved that successful outcome.

EXPENDITURES

As might be expected from the increases in the number of persons served and the number of persons rehabilitated, the expenditures in the program have also increased through the years (see Table 2.2).

TABLE 2.1

Number of Cases Served and Persons Rehabilitated by State VR Agencies, FY 1921-73

Fiscal Year	Cases Served	Persons Rehabilitated
1973	1,176,445	360,726
1972	1,111,045	326,138
1971	1,001,660	291,272
1970	875,911	266,975
1969	781,614	241,390
1968	680,415	207,918
1967	569,907	173,594
1966	499,464	154,279
1965	441,332	134,859
1964	399,852	119,708
1963	368,696	110,136
1962	345,635	102,377
1961	320,963	92,501
1960	297,950	88,275
1959	280,384	80,739
1958	258,444	74,317
1957	238,582	70,940
1956	221,128	65,640
1955	209,039	57,981
1954	211,219	55,825
1953	221,849	61,308
1952	228,490	63,632
1951	231,544	66,193
1950	225,724	59,597
1949	216,997	58,020
1948	191,063	53,131
1947	170,143	43,880
1946	169,796	36,106
1945	161,050	41,925
1944	145,059	43,997
1943	129,207	42,618
1942	91,572	21,757
1941	78,320	14,579
1940	65,624	11,890
1939	63,575	10,747
1938	63,666	9,844
1937	NA	11,091
1936	NA	10,338
1935	NA	9,422
1934	NA	8,062
1933	NA	5,613
1932	NA	5,592
1931	NA	5,184
1930	NA	4,605
1929	NA	4,645
1928	NA	5,012
1927	NA	5,092
1926	NA	5,604
1925	NA	5,825
1924	NA	5,654
1923	NA	4,530
1922	NA	1,898
1921	NA	523

Note: NA = not available.

Source: SRS, Caseload Statistics: State Vocational Rehabilitation Agencies (1973), Table I, p. 9.

TABLE 2.2

Expenditures of the Federal-State Program, FY 1921-73

Fiscal Year	Total	Percent Federal
1973	729,656	80.0[*]
1972	696,841	79.5[*]
1971	631,371	79.5
1970	557,706	76.2
1969	455,865	74.8
1968	377,646	74.8
1967	303,846	74.1
1966	213,639	67.7
1965	154,140	61.4
1964	133,259	61.7
1963	113,111	61.3
1962	101,390	61.1
1961	88,150	61.1
1960	78,711	61.2
1959	71,206	61.7
1958	63,727	61.8
1957	54,282	62.0
1956	46,221	62.4
1955	38,629	61.6
1954	35,366	64.9
1953	34,583	66.3
1952	32,689	67.7
1951	30,273	69.4
1950	29,347	69.3
1949	25,819	70.6
1948	24,569	72.1
1947	19,313	73.5
1946	13,749	72.7
1945	9,856	72.4
1944	6,372	63.6
1943	5,630	49.1
1942	5,205	49.1
1941	4,711	48.4
1940	4,108	48.0
1939	3,992	45.9
1938	3,862	46.4
1937	3,319	45.6
1936	2,603	47.2
1935	2,248	45.9
1934	2,080	44.0
1933	2,176	45.9
1932	2,186	45.7
1931	2,043	45.7
1930	1,700	43.5
1929	1,490	44.6
1928	1,541	42.4
1927	1,407	44.9
1926	1,274	45.5
1925	1,187	43.8
1924	1,243	44.4
1923	1,188	44.2
1922	736	42.4
1921	285	32.8

[*]Estimate.

Sources: SRS, Statistical History, Federal-State Program of Vocational Rehabilitation 1920-1969 (June 1970), Table 41, p. 67; SRS, State Vocational Rehabilitation Agency in Fiscal Year, annual, 1970-73.

In 1921 the program began with a total annual expenditure of $285,000, with roughly one-third of it coming from the federal government. At the beginning of World War II, the program expenditures were only $4 million per year, with sharing on a fifty-fifty basis. At the end of the war, expenditures began to increase, especially after the 1954 amendments broadened the scope of the program. By 1956, annual program expenditures were about $50 million a year, with nearly two-thirds of it now coming from the federal government. After 1962, program expenditures passed the $100 million mark, and in the 1970s a half billion dollars per year were being spent. It is estimated that total program expenditures today are nearly $800 million, of which about 80 percent comes from the federal government.

In addition to the basic support program that finances the services offered in the state agencies, the federal government allocates funds for research, R&D projects, and training programs (see discussion in Chapter 3). It might be noted that although research funds have declined in recent years, approximately $20 million per year has been allocated for R&D projects and research and training centers. In addition, approximately $30 million per year has been allocated for training purposes.

THE CHANGING CONCERNS OF THE
REHABILITATION AGENCIES

When the program began after World War I, its basic concern was with the injured. The VA was concerned with the returning veterans and their ability to get jobs in the labor market. The state agencies were concerned with the industrially injured, and an intimate relationship existed between the state worker's compensation programs and the VR agencies.

Because of this concern for the injured, it was natural that orthopedic disabilities would be an important portion of the case load. As late as 1945, 50 percent of the persons rehabilitated each year were classified as having orthopedic impairments, including amputation of limbs and impairment of limbs, back, head, or chest. By 1964 the percentage had declined to 35 percent, and by 1970 to approximately one-fifth of the case load. That fraction has declined slightly further since 1970.

Table 2.3 shows the trends in types of impairments rehabilitated—what is known in rehabilitation parlance as "disabling conditions." One particular significant change is the growth in the categories of mental illness, mental retardation, and other types of behavioral disorders. In 1945 mental illness, mental retardation, and epilepsy

TABLE 2.3

Percentage of Cases, by Major Disabling Condition of Persons Rehabilitated by
State Vocational Rehabilitation Agencies, Selected Fiscal Years, FY 1925-72

Fiscal Year	Total Rehabilitation	Orthopedic	Visual	Hearing	Mental Illness	Mental Retardation	Heart	Pulmonary Tuberculosis	Epilepsy
1925	100.0	74.2	6.8	0.3	NA	NA	NA	NA	NA
1930	100.0	75.6	6.8	3.5	NA	NA	NA	NA	NA
1935	100.0	72.5	7.3	7.4	NA	NA	1.7	5.0	NA
1940	100.0	69.1	7.5	9.4	NA	NA	2.7	7.7	NA
1945	100.0	50.0	11.8	7.5	3.2	0.3	4.3	6.3	0.8
1950	100.0	43.3	11.9	8.9	3.4	0.8	3.9	8.2	1.8
1955	100.0	40.3	11.4	6.5	3.5	0.9	4.4	11.3	2.1
1960	100.0	40.3	10.7	6.1	6.5	3.3	4.8	7.0	2.1
1965	100.0	34.0	9.7	6.0	13.6	7.6	4.1	3.2	2.1
1970	100.0	21.5	8.8	5.6	24.7	11.8	2.9	1.1	1.7
1971	100.0	20.6	8.6	5.2	27.1	11.3	2.7	0.8	1.5
1972	100.0	20.0	8.5	5.3	28.6	11.6	2.4	0.7	1.5

Note: NA = not available

Sources: SRS, Statistical History, Federal State Program of Vocational Rehabilitation 1920-69 (June 1970), Table 24, p. 47; SRS, "Information Memorandum RSA-IM-74-1," July 2, 1973, p. 3.

together comprised just about 4 percent of the number of rehabilitants.
The most dramatic increase came in the field of mental illness, which
by 1965 constituted nearly 14 percent of the case load and in 1970
nearly one-quarter of the case load. (In fiscal 1967 and later years,
drug addiction and alcoholism are treated as mental illness, certainly
accounting for part of the large increase.) Mental retardation also
showed a large percentage increase, starting with less than 1 percent
in 1945 and rising to 12 percent of the case load today.

The trend is significant for our purposes. Although orthopedic
disabilities are still prominent in terms of the total number of cases
served or the percentage of cases rehabilitated, the primary growth
has been in mental retardation, mental illness, and other related conditions. That growth has brought about a new rehabilitation interest
that is reflected in the research activity. In fact, more than a pro-
portionate amount of research funds have gone to the newer categories
of disabling conditions, a fact that will be manifested in our sample
of research reports.

There is yet another significance to the change in the case load.
The growth of the mental retardation category came in the Kennedy
years, when emphasis was placed on that condition classification.
When in the Johnson era the attention began to shift to the war on poverty, it became apparent that some of the poor suffered from behavioral disorders or from conditions that closely approximated them.
It was hypothesized that some techniques that had proved useful in
restoring persons with behavioral disorders might also be used to
restore persons who were culturally or socially disadvantaged.

Once social and cultural disadvantages came to be viewed as
handicaps that could be rehabilitated, the traditional goal of the
rehabilitation agencies, of placing a person in employment or in an
activity closely related to employment, came into question. Increased
functioning capacity, improvement of self-concept or ability to sustain
oneself in the activities of daily living began to be considered as
possible outcome measures. Similarly, as rehabilitation agencies
began to admit persons who suffered from drug addiction or alcoholism,
there were great pressures put upon them to redefine success in terms
other than restoration to the labor market.

NEW DIRECTIONS

We are in the midst of these trends, and it is difficult to tell
where they will end. The Vocational Rehabilitation Act of 1973 apparently signals some departure from emphasis on the socially and culturally disadvantaged. Congress has exhibited concern over the

individuals who are most severely handicapped and has mandated a study to identify those persons. Undoubtedly, that interest has been prompted by a feeling that the severely handicapped merit greater priority in the receipt of rehabilitation services. Whatever the outcome, that interest may mark a return to the more traditional concerns of rehabilitation agencies. However, the trends of the past two decades have left their impact on rehabilitation research, as the next chapter will confirm.

REFERENCES

Treitel, R. "Rehabilitation of the Disabled," Social Security Survey of the Disabled: 1966. U.S. Department of Health, Education, and Welfare, Social Security Administration, 1970.

U.S. Department of Health, Education, and Welfare, Social and Rehabilitation Service. Caseload Statistics: State Vocational Rehabilitation Agencies (1973).

____. State Vocational Rehabilitation Agency in Fiscal Year 1973.

____. State Vocational Rehabilitation Agency in Fiscal Year 1972.

____. State Vocational Rehabilitation Agency in Fiscal Year 1971.

____. State Vocational Rehabilitation Agency in Fiscal Year 1970.

____. Statistical History, Federal State Program of Vocational Rehabilitation 1920-1969 (June 1970).

____. Rehabilitation Services Administration. "Information Memorandum RSA-IM-74-1," July 2, 1973.

RESEARCH FUNDING

Most of the research with which we are concerned is funded by
the federal government—principally, by the Department of Health,
Education, and Welfare (HEW). Estimates for 1973 show HEW obli-
gating nearly $2 billion for research and development (NSF, 1972,
Table C-3). The breakdown of those funds among HEW agencies is
given in Table 3.1. It is interesting to note that only one-fifth of the
research funded is actually done intramurally, while more than one-
half is conducted by universities and colleges.[*]

Some portion of funding in every division of HEW is given over
to rehabilitation research. Undoubtedly, the major rehabilitation-
oriented divisions are SRS, the home of the joint state-federal rehabilitation programs, and NIH. The expenditures of SRS are primarily in
applied research, while NIH deals more with basic and developmental
projects.[†] The VA is also a major contributor to rehabilitation research. Although we are unable to distinguish rehabilitation research

---

[*] In 1971 out of total HEW obligations for research and development of nearly $1.5 billion, nearly $300 million was obligated for
intramural research and $769 million for research in universities
and colleges. Another $217 million was allocated for research done
by other nonprofit institutions (NSF, 1972, Table C-7, p. 62).

[†] See National Science Foundation, 1972, Appendix A, p. 39, for
definitions of those terms.

TABLE 3.1

Federal Funds for Total Research and Development, 1973
(millions of dollars)

Agency	Obligation (Est.)
Food and Drug Administration	56.5
Health Services and Mental Health	257.8
National Institute of Education Administration	125.0
National Institutes of Health	1,368.6
Office of Child Development	19.4
Office of Education	72.4
Social and Rehabilitation Service	45.0
Social Security Administration	12.6
Total HEW	1,957.2

Source: NSF, 1972, Table C-3, p. 54.

from other types of funded research, the VA's estimated R&D obligation for 1973 was $75.5 million. Almost all of the rehabilitation research conducted by the VA is done intramurally.

As shown in Table 3.2, the VR program expenditures for research have grown more than tenfold since the mid-1950s. Separate funds began to be appropriated for research only after the 1954 amendments mentioned below. From the point of view of the state rehabilitation agencies, R&D funds have a certain attractiveness. Research funds come to the state agencies virtually free. Apart from nominal cost-sharing arrangements, the state is not obliged to match those research funds. We will see that a large part of the funds are spent on R&D projects, some of which contain a large service component. Thus, from the point of view of the state agencies, funding an R&D project with 100 percent federal money is a relatively costless way of expanding services and, perhaps, of purchasing sorely needed equipment or hiring additional personnel. One of the recurring problems in our report on evaluation of rehabilitation research is that many of the projects that come under our review are labeled as research but are essentially service programs.

On the other hand, the state rehabilitation agencies may view with certain misgivings the funds allocated to research. Although the federal agencies clear with the states before funds are actually allocated, the state agencies have no direct control over the methods by which the funds are awarded. Moreover, state agencies may be fearful

TABLE 3.2

Federal Grants for VR Programs, 1955-73

Year	R&D	R&D as a Percentage of Program Expenditures	Training and Traineeships	Research and Training Centers
1955	299	0.8	637	—
1956	1,181	2.6	1,990	—
1957	2,000	3.7	2,668	—
1958	3,600	5.6	4,156	—
1959	4,600	6.5	4,651	—
1960	6,390	8.1	6,117	—
1961	8,163	9.3	7,106	—
1962	9,450	9.3	9,427	723
1963	10,994	9.7	12,108	1,700
1964	15,179	11.4	16,442	2,965
1965	17,069	11.1	19,770	4,084
1966	20,568	9.6	24,520	7,574
1967	21,015	6.9	29,717	8,575
1968	21,304	5.6	31,203	10,225
1969	21,425	4.7	31,702	10,275
1970	20,833	3.7	27,681	9,761
1971	17,234	2.7	32,698	10,274
1972	22,269	3.2	20,966	13,042
1973 (est.)	19,255	2.6	27,700	12,203

Sources: Larry L. Kiser, "Economic Efficiency and Public Vocational Rehabilitation Policy" (Ph.D. Dissertation, Rutgers University, 1973), Table 1, p. 16; SRS, State Vocational Rehabilitation Agency Fact Sheet Booklet, annual (1971-72).

of innovation and resist undertaking research that could lead to new
ideas, methods, or plans for rehabilitation. Evaluations of existing
methods of rehabilitation could call into question the validity of the
very practices that the agencies have been using. One final argument
against allocating funds to research is the notion that research funds
compete with program funds and that every dollar spent on research
detracts from funds for basic program support.

The battle for research funds is continuous. Although the long-
term growth is dramatic, recent years have shown slight declines in
absolute terms. We may attribute the declines to national budgetary
trends for R&D funds in general. As shown in Table 3.2, R&D funds
were 6 percent of program expenditures at the end of the 1950s. In
1964 they reached a high of 11.4 percent of program funds, and there-
after the proportions declined. In recent years research funds have
been averaging 3 percent of the amount allocated for basic program
support.

An overall view reveals that funding for SRS R&D as a percentage
of all HEW R&D had increased through 1969 to 3.45 percent, but in
recent years the amount has leveled off at 2.3 percent. Total NIH
funding has remained fairly constant at 69 percent of HEW R&D, but
we are unable to establish with certainty the proportion attributable
to rehabilitation research. Similarly, we cannot separate the portion
of VA research funding allocated to rehabilitation. In general, trends
indicate a fairly stable pattern of rehabilitation research relative to
all R&D.

MAJOR DEVELOPMENTS IN
REHABILITATION RESEARCH

Perhaps the earliest attempts to apply research techniques to
the rehabilitation process date back to the sixteenth century, when
Juan Paulo Bonet developed a manual alphabet for use by the deaf
(Garrett, 1969, pp. 34-35). By the middle of the seventeenth century
Germany had originated a wax tablet with raised figures for use by
the blind and was producing them on a widespread scale (Garrett,
1969, p. 56). Improvements in communication aids for the deaf and
blind continued through the eighteenth and nineteenth centuries. In
1850 Thomas Gallaudet brought the manual method for the deaf to the
United States. Louis Braille developed his method of communication
for the blind in the nineteenth century, but there was a regrettable
gap of time between the invention and its widespread acceptance and
use; it took nearly 40 years before the method was adopted in Britain
and the United States.

Medical treatment is an integral aspect of rehabilitation. The
hospital movement and the establishment of public health facilities
brought the need for physical restoration to the public's attention and
helped to promote the development of corrective methods. Not surprisingly, orthopedic surgery made great advances in the nineteenth
century (Obermann, 1965, p. 79). The problem posed by communi-
cable diseases encouraged scientific studies of their cause and cure.
We know for example, that concern for victims of the white plague in
the urban ghettos led to research in tuberculosis. Robert Koch identified the tubercule bacillus in 1882, but it was many years before his
research findings were translated into concrete programs of prevention
or treatment.

A major rehabilitation trend in this country has been a blend of
restorative and training aspects. As far back as 1848 there was an
experimental school for the training of persons identified as "idiots"
(a term for which we have since found a number of euphemisms).
Samuel Howe directed a study that led to the establishment in 1851 of
the Massachusetts School for Idiotic and Feeble Minded Youth.

The precedent for government intervention in research was set
in the field of agriculture in the middle and late nineteenth century.
The research approach of the Department of Agriculture and its closely
related land-grant colleges established under the Morrill Act in 1862
was a combination of the scientific and the practical. The first commissioner of agriculture, Isaac Newton, decided to investigate the
individual disciplinary components of agriculture (chemistry, botany,
and so forth) "along academic lines in the hope that the farmer would
gain increased awareness of his surroundings and indirectly obtain
higher production" (Dupree, 1957, p. 152). Such theoretical investigation met with public pressure to produce practical results. The
notion of demonstration projects, prominent in vocational rehabilitation
research, can be traced back to Seaman Knapp's experiences in establishing a demonstration farm to convince the farmers that seed selection, deep plowing and crop rotation would enable them to increase
productivity (Dupree, 1957, p. 181).

Private and governmental forces joined together in an attempt
to rehabilitate those wounded in World War I. The federal government
used a building in New York, donated by Jeremiah Millbank, as an
experimental laboratory for learning how to rehabilitate injured sol-
diers. Both the American Red Cross and the United States Army were
also concerned with the veterans. When the Red Cross recognized
that it could not fund care and rehabilitation of the disabled indefinitely,
its Institute for Crippled and Disabled Men was taken over by the

government. The institute was eventually incorporated into the federal veterans program and into the rehabilitation program after 1921.[*]

The advent of the settlement house and the social worker raised social consciousness about the problems of the poor and the disadvantaged. As far back as the turn of the century there were attempts to find the number of poor, the number of industrially injured, and similar measures of disability or want. The federal rehabilitation agency recognized the need for better information, but it was not until 1928 that the Federal Board for Vocational Education issued "A Study of Rehabilitated Persons: A Statistical Analysis of the Rehabilitation of 6319 Disabled Persons." The finding of that study, which sought to determine the relative merits of different methods of rehabilitation, was that half the rehabilitations that occurred were a result of training (Obermann, 1965, p. 258). That same year also saw an attempt by the federal board to estimate the average cost of vocational rehabilitation.

World War II provided another major impetus for rehabilitation research. War injuries stimulated research in prosthetics and orthopedics. Prominent advocates of the "team" rehabilitation approach, such as Kessler and Rusk, demonstrated the practical results of their efforts in armed forces hospitals. Both men continued their work after the war, when the civilian programs received boosts in funding.

The establishment of NIH following the war was intended to help develop a concentration in basic research. NIH also sought to stimulate interest in innovative research and to help shift research directions when conditions required (The Advancement of Knowledge, p. 2).

Another major change occurred in 1954 when amendments to the Vocational Rehabilitation Act called for the establishment of an R&D program. The driving force behind the program was Mary Switzer. She, along with others, had been convinced by the activity in both the medical and agricultural fields that research could make a practical contribution to rehabilitation. That goal became one of the criteria for proposal selection: Proposals were to be judged on how well they might extend and advance the knowledge and techniques necessary for successful vocational rehabilitation. That research program provided a major link between the government and private rehabilitation agencies such as the Easter Seal Organization and the various associations of the disabled. As the fields of inquiry broadened, cooperation became essential for optimal implementation of research results.

---

[*]Much of the information in this paragraph was gleaned from a conversation with Rudolph Clemens at the Red Cross National Headquarters.

Two additions to the basic R&D program occurred in 1961. The
Office of Vocational Rehabilitation began an international research
program, thereby expanding the areas in which research could be conducted. The expansion permitted not only an increased variety of
possible topics but also the wider dissemination of research results.
Another development in that same year was the introduction of research
and training centers: university-based facilities established to do
research and training. Those research centers focus on a specific
rehabilitation-related program, such as physical medicine, mental
retardation, or vocational rehabilitation.

THE CURRENT SITUATION

We shall now focus upon the procedures used in SRS, the major
government agency responsible for research specifically oriented
toward rehabilitation. Although other agencies—VA, NIH, and the
Social Security Administration (SSA), for example—deal with the subject, it is SRS that is responsible for initiating major policy changes
regarding rehabilitation. [*] Hence, it is through an examination of this
agency that we can gain the fullest appreciation of developments in
rehabilitation research.

Proposal Selection

The Social and Rehabilitation Service was established in 1967
to incorporate a number of existing bureaus under a single administrator. One of the bureaus moved to SRS was the Office of Vocational
Rehabilitation (OVR), which was subsequently renamed the Rehabilitation Service Administration (RSA). [†]

---

[*] Prior to 1956 SSA had very little input into rehabilitation
research. In 1956 cooperative research and demonstration projects
were authorized by Section 1110, Title XI, of the amended Social
Security Act. Another part of the R&D program of SRS is the Social
Services Research and Demonstrations, which is also funded in part
by Section 1110. A third influence of SSA on SRS began in 1963 with
Section 1115, which authorized demonstration projects in public
assistance.

[†] The OVR, which had existed in one form or another since 1921,
was established in the Federal Security Agency in 1943 and had been
a part of HEW since 1953.

From 1955 to 1970 the funds for R&D grants were allocated through in-house planning in Washington. Applications were reviewed on the basis of the soundness of a proposal and its relevancy to the budget priorities of SRS (or its previous counterpart). Since the budget structure was relatively loose, funds could be shifted between disability classes. Applications were then approved or rejected according to recommendations made by expert members of one of the four study sections: medicine, psychosocial, sensory, and general. After the preliminary stage, proposals were sent to the National Advisory Council. Once the council had rated the application, the final decision was made by the administrator of SRS.

After several agency attempts to revise the structure, a more complete change in the system was undertaken in order to streamline the grant procedure by eliminating delays and accelerating the processing of applications. The study sections were discontinued, and the National Advisory Council's role was changed from one of proposal review to one of passing on the general issues for study. Applications are currently reviewed in-house by SRS technical experts. In line with the present federal administration's desire for an expanded role by states in the expenditure of federal funds, consideration is given to comments from both regional staff and state agencies regarding individual applications. Applications must offer assurance that the project will be valuable, that an adequate staff exists to administer it, and that some acceptable strategy has been developed for its implementation. An estimate of expenses and a cost-saving proposal must also be included.

SRS continues to develop new strategies for the allocation of research funds. In order to direct future research more closely, strategies are being developed to allocate money on the basis of issues, state of the art, and those disability areas where research is most needed. The hope is that once SRS has identified problem areas, researchers will respond with proposals directed to those areas.

As noted above, even the "new" funding system is undergoing change. The 1973 legislation calls for rehabilitation research to shift from the SRS to the RSA; the commissioner of RSA, rather than the SRS administrator, will have final authority on application approval.

The study-section procedure, presumably abandoned by SRS, has continued as an integral part of the funding procedures at NIH, where grant applications are assigned to one of several special study units for review. Those sections consist of 10 to 15 qualified consultants, each of whom reviews a fraction of the total reports and then writes a detailed appraisal. The reviewer rates the importance of the research problem, originality of approach, competence of researchers, experimental design, facilities, and budget. Applications approved by the study section are then rated. After aggregating

and normalizing the various scores, a priority listing is established.
Then the information is forwarded to one of the national advisory coun-
cils (there is one for each of the grant-awarding units in NIH) for final
consideration. The council's decision to approve or disapprove is
based upon a review of program relevance, needs of the particular
institute, the need for new research in an area, and so on.

The VA also has a peer-review system, which seems appropriate in that most of its research is intramural. The review is usually
conducted by the research and education committee of the hospital.
(In cases requiring special consideration, a proposal can be sent to
the central VA office for merit review.) The amount of funded research
at a particular hospital is based on an in-hospital review of likely needs.
The information is then forwarded to Washington for approval.

In 1962, in an effort to offer researchers access to various
techniques, specialized help, and/or necessary information, the VA
established four regional support centers. Those centers provide
individual researchers with interdisciplinary assistance in formulating
and conducting medical research. The assistance takes the form of
information on research design, preparation of statistical techniques
and mathematical models, scientific data preparation and management,
computer programming, and identification and location of special
resources (VA, 1969, p. 3).

Program Research in SRS

In addition to the R&D program discussed above, SRS has three
formats for the conduct of rehabilitation research: the Regional
Research Institutes in Social Welfare (RRI), the Regional Rehabilitation Research Institute (RRRI), and Research and Training Centers
(R&T Centers). Those agencies are built around various areas of
socially-oriented care. Since the institutes and centers received
continuous funding to research specific areas, they have been able
to build a staff of professional specialists. Moreover, the location of
the institutes within universities enables them to draw upon the resources of a number of experts from a variety of disciplines.

R&T Centers do more than pursue research. They conduct
training programs for rehabilitation personnel and service programs
for those in need of rehabilitation. In addition, they help to coordinate
their own special research efforts with those of regional, state, and
private agencies. The RRIs are responsible for providing direction
to the states regarding operational research problems. The RRRIs
conduct and publish "state of the art" studies so that both the SRS and
the public are kept informed of current developments.

A number of problems have surfaced with regard to the institutes. Their funding has been criticized as insufficient for achievement of stated objectives. Some have noted that SRS sometimes intervenes, changing emphasis and priorities in mid-year, thereby creating planning problems. In addition, the RRIs' research objective has often been subordinated to technical assistance for state VR agencies, and there has been a trend away from client-oriented research to service-delivery research. But viewed as a whole, the difficulties encountered by those programmatic agencies have really been natural growing pains; we can now anticipate a stage where such agencies can mature and prosper.

Research Utilization

The topic of research utilization has become very important in recent years. Much research has been done in the past 20 years, but has it been put to use? SRS began considering and implementing a research-utilization branch in the late 1960s. Abstracts of the final reports of all SRS projects were prepared and disseminated over the next few years. As an experiment, nine research-utilization specialists have been designated to operate out of VR agencies; their function is to serve as a liaison between research and practice. SRS has also established two research-utilization laboratories responsible for adapting research results for practical application and for disseminating effective research results. The utilization of research must continue to be a high priority, for it is only through such usage that our ultimate goals can be achieved.

Successful research utilization programs may create feedback that researchers can use to improve the methodological adequacy and policy utility of their work. SRS has apparently recognized that possibility and requires recipients of its R&D grants to include a research-utilization strategy in their plans.

SUMMARY

We have seen how the combination of periods of need (e.g., World Wars I and II) and intensely dedicated people has served to produce a rehabilitation-research program. Government has played a major role in the development—a role that is constantly changing. Continued improvements are likely as the efforts of researchers, practitioners, and government officials focus upon reducing both the cost of rehabilitation and the duration of an individual's handicap.

The following chapters review and synthesize the attempts of various researchers in a number of disciplines with a variety of techniques to develop better rehabilitation methods. Our panel members have tried to point out the methodological strengths and weaknesses and the degree of policy utility found in their samples of research.

REFERENCES

Allen, E. M. "Why Are Research Grants Applications Disapproved?" _Science_ 132 (November 1960), pp. 1532-34.

Dupree, A. H. _Science in the Federal Government_. Cambridge: The Belknap Press of Harvard University Press, 1957.

Eaves, G. N. "Who Reads Your Project Grant Application to the National Institute of Health?" Federation Proceedings. Washington, D.C.: National Institutes of Health, 1972.

Garrett, J. F. "Historical Background." _The VR of the Disabled_, D. Malikin and H. Rusalem, eds. New York: Union Press, 1969, pp. 29-38.

Havelock, R. G. "Translating Theory into Practice." In _Rehabilitation Record_. Washington, D.C.: Government Printing Office, 1969.

ICD Rehabilitation and Research Center, S. G. DiMichael, project director. "A Research Utilization Laboratory Comprehensive Rehabilitation Center." Unpublished, New York, N.Y., the Center, 1973.

Kessler, H. H. _The Crippled and Disabled: Rehabilitation of the Physically Handicapped in the United States_. New York: Columbia University Press, 1935.

Kiser, L. K. "Economic Efficiency and Public Vocational Rehabilitation Policy." Ph.D. dissertation, Rutgers University, 1973.

Kunce, J. T. _The Roles and Function of a Regional Rehabilitation Research Institute_, Research Series No. 8. Columbia, Mo.: Regional Rehabilitation Research Institute, University of Missouri, 1973.

Magno, J. B., U.S. Department of Health, Education, and Welfare, Social and Rehabilitation Service. Letter to authors, April 2, 1974.

Moriarty, J. "Special Issue Announcing P*E*V*R*S*." Rehabilitation Tomorrow 3, no. 9 (December 1973), pp. 1-2.

National Easter Seal Society for Crippled Children and Adults. "1974 Facts about Easter Seals." Chicago, 1974.

National Rehabilitation Association. "Testimony of the National Rehabilitation Association at Oversight Hearings Conducted by Select Education Subcommittee of House Committee on Education and Labor." Mimeographed. Washington, D.C., April 1974.

National Science Foundation. Data Book. Washington, D.C.: the Foundation, 1973.

_____. Federal Funds for Research Development and Other Scientific Activities, vol. 21. Washington, D.C.: Government Printing Office, 1972.

Obermann, C. E. A History of Vocational Rehabilitation in America. Minneapolis: Denison, 1965.

Paralyzed Veterans of America, Inc. "Paralyzed Veterans of America." Washington, D.C.: the Organization.

Pelz, D., and Andrews, F. Scientists in Organizations. New York: Wiley, 1966.

Rogers, E. "Research Utilization in Rehabilitation." Rehabilitation Psychology, W. Neff, ed. Washington, D.C.: American Psychological Association, 1971.

Rotundo, A. "The SRS System for Project Grants," Human Needs 1, no. 8 (February 1973).

Rusalem, H. "The Research Role." The VR of the Disabled, D. Malikin and H. Rusalem, eds. New York: Union Press, 1969, pp. 155-69.

Rusk, H., and Taylor, J. New Hope for the Handicapped. New York: Harper & Row, 1946.

Scott, R. The Making of Blind Men. New York: Russell Sage Foundation, 1969.

Simmons, J. S., ed. Public Health in the World Today. Cambridge,
     Mass.: Harvard University Press, 1949.

Sussman, M., ed. Sociology and Rehabilitation. Washington, D.C.:
     American Sociological Association, 1965.

Switzer, M. E. "Legislative Contributions." The VR of the Disabled,
     D. Malikin and H. Rusalem, eds. New York: Union Press,
     1969, pp. 39-53.

True, A. C. A History of Agricultural Experimentation and Research
     in the United States 1607-1925. Washington, D.C.: Government
     Printing Office, 1937.

U.S. Department of Health, Education, and Welfare, Public Health
     Service. Grants for Research Projects, policy statement.
     Washington, D.C.: Government Printing Office, 1972.

_____. The Advancement of Knowledge for the Nation's Health. Wash-
     ington, D.C.: Government Printing Office.

U.S. Department of Health, Education, and Welfare, Social and
     Rehabilitation Services. State Vocational Rehabilitation Agency
     Fact Sheet Booklet, Fiscal Year 1972. Washington, D.C.:
     Rehabilitation Services Administration, December 1972.

_____. State Vocational Rehabilitation Agency Fact Sheet Booklet, Fiscal
     Year 1971. Washington, D.C.: Rehabilitation Services Admin-
     istration, January 1972.

_____. Proceedings of a Workshop, I. Robinault and M. Weisinger, eds.
     Washington, D.C.: Government Printing Office, March 1971.

Veterans Administration. Administrator of Veterans Affairs, annual
     report. Washington, D.C.: Government Printing Office, 1973.

_____. Medical Research in the Veterans Administration, annual report.
     Washington, D.C.: Government Printing Office, 1969.

Williams, R. C. The United States Public Health Service 1798-1950.
     Washington, D.C.: Public Health Service, 1951.

Wright, G., and Trotter, A. B. Rehabilitation Research. Madison,
     Wis.: University of Wisconsin, 1968.

REHABILITATION
AND SOCIAL WORK

This chapter focuses on studies involving the profession of social work or social-welfare agencies in the rehabilitation of the disabled and handicapped. Broadly conceived, social work is concerned with the provision of a range of resources to individuals, groups, and communities in order to prevent social dysfunction and to enhance positive social functioning. Historically, the thrust of social work has been toward improving the social functioning of individuals. While the 1960s witnessed a reorientation of social-work activity toward larger social units as targets of intervention, there can be no gainsaying the necessity for continued efforts aimed at the social rehabilitation of individuals who have been dislocated by any number of social-functioning impairments.

Whether the source of an individual's handicap is physical, psychological, or social, there is always a social expression of disability. The individual's role in the world of work, in formal and informal community participation, in family-related activities, and in the conduct of everyday life may all be involved. And because role impairments are differentially sanctioned by society, their impact on an individual's self-image must clearly be reckoned with.

The types of activities devoted to rehabilitation are as manifold as the causes and expressions of disability. Even though social work does not deal directly with the medical and physical restorative dimensions of rehabilitation or with vocational rehabilitation per se, its focus on facilitating social functioning can involve practically all of

---

This chapter was written by Bruce Lagay, Associate Professor of Social Work, Graduate School of Social Work, Rutgers University.

TABLE 4.1

Range of Handicaps and Clients Addressed in Rehabilitation
Studies Involving Social Work

Disability	Number of Studies
Mental illness	9
Various disabilities of public-assistance clients	7
Mental retardation	7
Various chronic illnesses and disabilities of the young and the old	7
Alcoholism	6
Social disabilities of public offenders	6
Other disabilities and handicaps[*]	6
Total	48

[*]Cardiac and circulatory diseases, 1; drug abuse, 1; renal
disease, 1; respiratory diseases, 1; visual impairments, 2.

Source: Compiled by the authors.

an individual's institutionally-defined relationships. Social workers
carrying out rehabilitation functions most often find themselves dealing
with the family and community social functioning of their clients. On
yet another level of intervention, social workers are with increasing
frequency engaged in the planning of services and the organization of
communities in support of service development. Thus, when examining
the involvement of social work in the area of rehabilitation, one must
not only consider the full range of handicaps by virtue of their social
dimension, but the various levels of intervention with both client and
nonclient target groups as well. The range of handicaps and clients
addressed in our 48 social-work-related studies is illustrated in
Table 4.1.

Studies from several of the categories in Table 4.1 will be considered in other chapters where their specific mode of intervention is
even more pertinent. For example, studies dealing with the rehabilitation of public assistance clients will be assessed in the chapter on
program coordination (Chapter 12), since all of them focus on coordination of service between vocational-rehabilitation and social-welfare
agencies. Substantively treated elsewhere as well are studies dealing
with the rehabilitation of public offenders (Chapter 7).

For reasons that will become apparent shortly, the assessment
of the research and policy utility of the studies reviewed here should
be of greater interest to applied and evaluation researchers and to

federal research and evaluation policy formulators than to practitioner and planners in the substantive areas studied.

QUALITY OF THE RESEARCH UNDERTAKEN

The assessment of the overall quality of research in the studies reviewed represents a composite rating of a number of dimensions: research design, hypothesis formulation, sampling procedures, and data analysis. The types of design can be broadly divided as follows: 26 nonexperimental, 21 experimental, and one unclassified. However, the majority of the "experimental" designs (13 out of 21) were technically preexperimental in character (see Campbell and Stanley, 1973). Nineteen of the 26 nonexperimental designs were subclassified as demonstrations. Only five of the total of 48 studies were true experimental designs; under the most rigorous standards, only those five could be argued to be internally valid. However, to judge internal validity exclusively in terms of the presence of a true experimental design would be to apply an uncommonly stringent standard for the assessment of evaluative research where the appropriateness of quasi-experimental design features are commonly accepted. Hence, in judging the internal validity of quasi-experimental designs, we take into consideration the researcher's awareness of alternative hypotheses, even though they may not have gone so far as to test them, and their utilization of sampling procedures that, although nonrandom, are rigorously stated and adhered to.

Yet even with the most lenient of standards, the general picture of the quality of research reviewed is not good. For example, it is disheartening to observe that on the matter of hypothesis formulation nearly one-third (N = 15) of all the studies reviewed either failed to state a hypothesis (N = 9) or stated it in a vague or untestable form (N = 6). Furthermore, only 24 studies—half of those reviewed—mentioned alternative hypotheses, and only 12 of those went so far as to test those alternative hypotheses. External influences on the study were mentioned in only 21 of the 48 studies, and only 25 of the 48 made mention of internal influences, such as staff selection and motivation on the experimental input.

With reference to sampling, only a small group of studies (N = 5) employed any form of random sampling. Given the understandable constraints on ability to random sample, it is all the more incumbent upon researchers meticulously to account for the screening-in procedures and attrition of sample members. In only 11 studies was it possible to follow the studies' total <u>N</u>s through various intake, process, and outcome categories over time and not lose cases for unexplained reasons.

The statistical analyses of findings were elementary. A majority of the studies (N = 28) restricted themselves to simple descriptive statistics. As for associational analysis, five studies employed chi square, eight studies employed the t test, and two employed the F test to establish statistical significance. Multivariate analysis was used in four cases.

Given these contributing conditions, it should not be surprising that on the ten-point rating scale of overall quality of research methodology, only two studies received a rating of ten. Seven studies rated eight or nine; ten rated six or seven; 29 rated five or less.

Among the relatively more adequate studies (those receiving a rating of eight or more), three came from the area of mental retardation; two each came from the disability areas of mental illness and disabled public assistance clients; one each came from the areas of public offenders and the "other disabilities and handicaps" category. The two disability categories not represented in the above group are "alcoholics" and "chronic illnesses and disabilities of the young and of the old." Alcoholism is a particularly difficult disability to research, especially in the follow-up stage—a design feature all six of the alcoholism studies read attempted to include. While none of the alcohol studies attained an above-8 rating, as a category they had the highest average research rating. A similar performance was not observed for the category of chronic illness and disabilities.

The more adequate studies seemed invariably to be conducted by either university-based investigators or by researchers working out of large national organizations.

Four of the nine studies attempted rather complex predictive efforts with fairly sophisticated data handling (Sue and Wippel, 1971; Armatas et al., 1970; Sells, 1967; Parnicky and Kahn, 1963). One of these four (Armatas et al., 1970), and two other studies (Daniels et al., 1970; Habif, 1968) dealt with complex institutional/organizational designs. The penultimate study, one of the most creative reviewed, reorganized a ward of chronic psychiatric patients into a problem-solving group devoted to developing employment services, an industrial workshop, and eventually community housing. Three studies (Long and Fontana, 1973; Pagan, 1968; Selling and Gaza, 1967) presented straightforward and relatively competently executed program-evaluation designs.

The phrase "relatively adequate studies" is used advisedly. The features that commend them are usually their candor and sophistication in recognizing their own shortcomings. The following demonstration of the rehabilitation of emotionally disabled, institutionalized individuals is an example of this phenomenon:[*]

---

[*]Edited from SRS abstract of Armatas et al., 1970, by G. Spencer (RD-1457).

From a potential population of 1,385 domiciliary residents, 282 were referred to the program and a total of 64 chronically institutionalized men with a variety of disabilities voluntarily participated in a program that lasted 12 months. The program consisted of daily attendance at vocational training sessions utilizing T-group techniques, self-governing dormitory living, individualized and group counseling, job placement and follow-up. Training expenses and a small stipend were provided. Dependent variables were completion of the program and independent functioning in a job in a noninstitutionalized setting. Independent variables included an extensive battery of psychological measures as well as traditional sociodemocratic histories.

Thirty-two men completed the program and the other half dropped out. Only 15 men were considered a "total success" achieving independent functioning in the community. Only five men hold jobs for which they were actually trained. Few of the independent measures predicted program success. The most significant finding was that participants who showed initial feelings of weakness, dependency and conformity had higher rates of success than those who were initially dominant and assertive. It was suggested that the central thesis was not the building of independence, but the transfer of dependency from institutional settings to community settings.

The SRS abstract from which that material is summarized states:

Although the preface to the project's final report suggests that it is a model program that has achieved impressive results, this is not supported by the data. The monograph, however, is well worth reading. The development of a theoretical rationale for the program is extensively and clearly developed. It brings together a wide range of interdisciplinary thought on the problems of rehabilitation. Additionally, the report is an honest one. The body of the report does not gloss over failures but discusses them openly and with insight. The problems in utilizing commercial vocational training programs and the resistance of clients to sensitivity training is documented well. The central thesis that institutional dependency can be transferred to a community setting that will allow dependent individuals to function in noninstitutionalized settings is compelling and encourages further investigation.

In summarizing the quality of research in the 48 studies examined, it should be noted that while assessment criteria and standards appropriate to quasi-experimental demonstration research were employed, only nine studies rated eight or higher on the ten-point scale provided. Failure to state testable hypotheses or any at all (N = 15), to recognize alternative hypotheses (N = 24), to report unambiguously screening procedures and sample attrition (N = 37), and incomplete data analysis contributed to the observed limitations in quality.

POLICY UTILITY

The policy-utility ratings of the studies reviewed were higher than their research-quality ratings. While only one study received a rating of ten, 13 studies rated eight or nine; ten studies, six or seven; 24 studies rated less than five. Those relatively higher policy ratings reflected our decision to recognize the potential utility of policy ideas, even where the accompanying research fell short of demonstrating technical validity.

None of the policy conclusions listed below will be particularly surprising to practitioners or planners, since most of the studies from which they are drawn are five to ten years old by now. Familiar instrumental themes abound—e.g., community-based versus institutional care for all categories of the disabled; coordination of related service delivery systems; outreach to previously unserved clients; consumer and client involvement in the development of services. Despite the justifiable criticism of prediction after the fact, we present the following notable policy notions, culled from the studies we have reviewed:

- Making accessible and assuring the delivery of health and welfare services to the disabled elderly (Gifford, 1968)
- Using the halfway house for public offenders returning to the community (O'Connor et al., 1973)
- Employing extended aftercare in the treatment of alcoholics (Pokorny et al., 1973)
- Involving Model Cities parents of the retarded in shaping services for their children (Long and Fontana, 1973)
- Coordinating social welfare and vocational rehabilitation services for public assistance clients (Pagan, 1968; Selling and Gaza, 1967)
- Holding onto potential dropouts among the educationally disadvantaged in public schools (Hayes, 1966)
- Using a task-focused milieu treatment for chronic psychiatric patients (Daniels et al., 1967)

The following abstract, edited from a summary of the last project's final report (Daniels et al. , 1970), provides an example of a study that received high ratings in terms of both quality of research and policy utility:

> The basic goal of the project was to reorganize a 30-bed male ward in a veterans hospital into a problem-solving organization of task groups requiring a division of labor and interdependence among patients and staff. A nonprofit corporation was formed for the delivery of psychiatric services in which patients participated on multiple levels including corporate directorships, management, and therapy. The initial task group was a patient-staff operated employment service. Subsequently, other task groups were added which included a patient-staff treatment planning and progress team, an industrial workshop and community housing.
>
> Typically, the patients in the project were in their early forties, had several previous hospitalizations, showed poor and unstable work records, were alienated from significant others and the normal sustaining network of relations, experienced a basic unhappiness with life and high levels of emotional distress, and had multiple serious psychiatric diagnoses.
>
> Although evaluative data cover a time before the industrial workshop and community housing were developed, they showed generally favorable results when compared to an active independent control group.
>
> A 12-18 month follow-up showed 44 percent less accumulated rehospitalization for the program; better work outcome (e.g., 136.5 compared to 115.3 equivalent 8-hour days worked on the average during the first 360 days after discharge, and 270.3 compared to 136.4 days worked on the first full-time job); and total cost savings of $3.30 per patient-day, of which $1.28 was a direct saving for the hospital. On the other hand, patients in the control therapeutic community program showed greater symptom improvement, a finding which could be attributed to the control ward's somewhat lower expectations and stress. In addition, approximately two-thirds of the patients from both groups had required rehospitalization at some time during the 18-month follow-up. These high relapse rates . . . led to the development of community housing and efforts to transfer the program into the community.

SUMMARY AND RECOMMENDATIONS

We have examined the quality of research and the policy utility
of 48 rehabilitation studies involving social work. Nine rated eight or
higher on methodological adequacy; 14 rated in the upper fifth of the
policy-utility scale.

The wide range of disabilities addressed, as well as the targets
and modes of intervention employed, resulted in a somewhat perfunc-
tory treatment of substantive policy issues. Eight studies of recognized
policy utility were identified, but an intensive assessment of their
future payoff would obviously entail more exhaustive efforts by experts
in each area of concern. Further summary comments are therefore
focused on matters of research methodology and their implications
for evaluative policy.

The correspondence between quality of research and policy utility
was not high. While six of the nine studies that rated eight or higher on
the quality-of-research scale also rated eight or higher on the policy-
utility scale, eight of the 14 studies rating eight or higher on policy
utility rated below eight on quality of research. The three research
studies of relatively high rating that were rated beneath eight on policy
utility were elaborate predictive studies that, while technically acceptable research efforts, did not make any positive policy contribution.

Since it was found that 85 percent of the studies (N = 39) were
evaluated by the individuals involved in delivering the programs
assessed, and since it was also observed that the more adequately
conducted studies were undertaken by university-based researchers
or researchers from large national organizations, it may not be
unreasonable to suggest that many of the less adequate studies lacked
the guidance of experienced evaluative researchers. Because it would
seem that two quite different sets of skills are involved in designing a
study and preparing a proposal and then actually spending months in
the field executing the design and later analyzing the data, it may be
advisable to look beyond study proposals in attempting to judge a
group's ability to produce valid research. Perhaps granting agencies
need to "walk" applicants through, or simulate with applicants, the
field execution of their submitted designs emphasizing the maintenance
of design validity and of complete analysis and reporting. An alternative arrangement might be to have research components of local
agency-initiated efforts carried out by institutional centers of proven
ability to produce quality research.

We have one final comment. Because of its concern with efficiency, as well as with the effectiveness of program, policy research
should employ elements of benefit-cost analysis. Historically,
rehabilitation research has been relatively more mindful of that

concern than have other human services. All future human services research ought to incorporate that essential feature.

REFERENCES

Those reports with an asterisk were included in our sample of 477 projects. A complete list of all reports reviewed by the author is available through the Bureau of Economic Research, Rutgers University.

*Armatas, J. P., et al. Rehabilitation of the Chronically Institutionalized. Lawrence, Kans.: Wadsworth Veterans Administration Center, University of Kansas, 1970.

Campbell, D. T., and Stanley, J. C. Experimental and Quasi-Experimental Designs for Research. Chicago: Rand McNally, 1973.

*Daniels, D. N., Fox, P. D., and Kuldav, J. M. The In-Vivo Therapeutic Community Through Task Groups. Stanford, Calif.: Stanford University School of Medicine, 1970.

*Gifford, A. Final Evaluation Report on Operation Reason: A Demonstration Project Designed to Develop Methods for Helping Elderly. Baltimore, Md.: Health and Welfare Council of the Baltimore Area, Inc., 1968.

*Habif, R. A. A Coordinated Program of Vocational Rehabilitation and Special Education Services for the Retarded. Boston: Massachusetts Rehabilitation Commission, 1968.

*Hayes, L. K. "Holding Power for Rehabilitation." Unpublished final report, Oklahoma City Schools, Oklahoma City, Okla., 1966.

*Long, E. L., and Fontana, L. A Final Report on Project STAR [Serving to Advance Rehabilitation]. New York: National Urban League, Family Service Association of America, National Association for Retarded Children, 1973.

*O'Connor, M. J., Dewing, J., and Frasier, C. Boston Offenders Service Project. Boston: Massachusetts Half-Way Houses, Inc., 1973.

*Pagan, A. <u>Vocational Rehabilitation of Disabled Public Welfare Clients</u>. Rio Piedras, P.R.: Division of Vocational Rehabilitation, 1968.

*Parnicky, J. J., and Kahn, H. <u>Evaluating and Developing Vocational Potential of Institutionalized Retarded Adolescents</u>. Bordentown, N.J.: Edward R. Johnstone Training and Research Center, 1963.

*Pokorny, A. D., Miller, B. A., Kanas, T., and Valles, J. "Effectiveness of Extended Aftercare in the Treatment of Alcoholism." <u>Quarterly Journal of Studies on Alcohol</u> 34 (1973): 435-43.

*Selling, L. L., and Gaza, C. T. <u>Vocational Rehabilitation of Disabled Public Assistance Clients</u>. Trenton, N.J.: New Jersey Rehabilitation Commission, 1967.

Sells, S. B., et al. <u>A Pilot Study of a Group of Narcotic Addicts One Year After Discharge</u>. Fort Worth: Texas Christian University, Institute of Behavioral Research, 1967.

*Sue, L., and Wippel, R. R. <u>The Alcoholic Offender</u>. Portland, Ore.: Multnomah County, 1971.

The first section of this chapter reviews a somewhat heterogeneous group of 28 studies, some of which are specifically covered in this chapter and in the subsequent chapter on adolescents. The handicaps in the sample were preponderantly in the area of mental illness (N = 15) and mental retardation (N = 4). The two most common settings for the studies were private rehabilitation centers, homes, societies, and so forth (25 percent), and VA hospitals (21.4 percent). Generally, the studies yielded interpretable and useful results: 19 of the reports were judged to be economically, ethically, and organizationally feasible.

Most of the findings were consistent with other research literature in the field. However, although 77.6 percent (N = 21) had well-defined hypotheses, only 22.4 percent (N = 7) presented alternative hypotheses; slightly more than half (53.8 percent) of the studies yielded data that were immediately suitable for application.

Of the studies that proved nonapplicable, a major reason for their unsuitability was poor methodology (35.3 percent—a figure that may have been inflated by our evaluation of a number of studies without benefit of sufficient technical reports). Another 29.4 percent of the studies focused on a limited population, thereby precluding any generalizations about other populations.

Since almost all of the studies (96.3 percent) were evaluated by people who were themselves in the programs, there exists the strong possibility of experimental bias. And doubts were raised by the check-

---

This chapter was written by Paul Lehrer, Assistant Professor of Psychiatry, Rutgers Medical School—CMDNJ.

listers about the ethical feasibility of repeating 15 percent of the
studies—those utilizing questionable behavior-modification techniques.
Although this reviewer tends to agree with several of their reservations, he is generally more positive about the ethical feasibility of the
studies.

Nearly three-quarters of the studies were based on an experimental design. The two most common designs were pretest/posttest
with control group and the one-shot case study. Although a number of
studies sorely needed control groups, careful use of contingency
reversal paradigms and multiple baselines (see Baer, 1968; Sidman,
1960) added to the validity of one-shot case studies. The variables
that were most frequently controlled for were type of disability (42.8
percent), age (33.1 percent), and sex (25 percent). Where strong
controls were not applied, the variables that were most commonly
considered were age (35.7 percent) and sex (39.3 percent).

All the studies reviewed come under the general category of
"behavior modification." A precise definition of the area is particularly difficult to establish, since all rehabilitation involves some use
of behavior-modification techniques. For example, any educational
program using "motivational materials" relies on a behavioral technique called "natural" or "inherent reinforcement"; any institution
that uses seclusion, locked wards, and so on, is using "time out";
any program that uses work for pay is using "token reinforcement";
any project that delimits a series of small steps between chronic
institutionalization and completely independent life is using "fading of
prompts"; any teaching program that provides small bits of information, to which students respond and are subsequently provided feedback, is using "programmed instruction."

This review will thus be restricted to studies that deal deliber-
ately with the evaluation of specific techniques of behavior modification.
It is written from the viewpoint of the behaviorally-oriented psychologist. We shall focus on the degree to which specific techniques are
effective, as well as on the effectiveness of overall rehabilitation
programs. Since the studies are generally of theoretical as well as
practical interest, their usefulness extends not only to behavioral
psychologists but to practitioners and administrators of institutional
and community-based programs. Table 5.1 summarizes the disabilities covered in the reports under review here.

The majority of the studies evaluated programs using token
reinforcement or some other variety of positive reinforcement. Originated by Ayllon and Azrin (1968) in their experimental work with
chronically psychotic female inpatients, that technique was later
extended to a more comprehensive rehabilitation program for chronically psychotic VA patients by Atthowe and Krasner (1968). It
currently has widespread and varied applications. Central to the

TABLE 5.1

Behavior-Modification Studies, by Type of Disability

Type of Disability	Number of Studies
Chronic mental illness	2
Delinquency	2
Retardation/neurological impairment	2
School dropouts	2
Geriatric infirmities	1
Alcoholism	1
Blindness	1

technique is the payment to clients of token reinforcement—tokens or points—for engaging in behaviors that approximate the goals of rehabilitation. In other words, it provides incentives for clients who are not motivated to improve by themselves. Among the prime candidates for token reinforcement are chronically institutionalized clients who have fully adopted the passive roles to which they have been socialized in institutional settings and hardcore delinquents, schizophrenics, and dropouts, who have forsworn the usual rewards of society (money, prestige, and so forth), because they appear to be unattainable, because socialization has taught them to obtain their rewards in deviant ways, because they have been punished for conforming to social values, or because they have internal psychological conflicts that prevent them from engaging in "normal" success-seeking behavior.

An additional function of token reinforcement is that of a "signal." For example, whenever the client engages in "healthy" behavior, something good happens, in turn helping him to discriminate healthy from sick behaviors. That is particularly important for retarded clients, whose use of language is not sufficiently developed for them to make the connections verbally. It is also important in institutional settings that are geared to custodial care rather than to active rehabilitation. Token reinforcement programs have a significant impact on staff behavior: They focus staff attention upon client behaviors that are relevant to rehabilitation, rather than on behavior whose purpose is to draw attention to the client. With the existence of tokens, small signs of behavioral improvement must be acknowledged and rewarded.

We shall not attempt to review the voluminous literature on token reinforcement. Suffice it to say that the technique is very effective in altering a variety of behaviors in "total institutions," and that it is also quite effective in partial institutions (e.g., schools, drop-in

centers, halfway houses, and so on) and in families. Where token
programs do not produce the desired results, their failure is attributable to difficulties in selecting target behaviors and in transferring
these behaviors to the outside world. For example, the target behaviors may entail the clients' continuing docility and conformity to institutional routines (Winnett and Winkler, 1972), or the token reinforcement system may not be designed to follow the person after discharge.[*]
The majority, which provide no such continuous follow-up, should be
designed to phase the client out gradually, in small steps that approximate life in the "real world" (Atthowe, 1973).

Legal opinion is also beginning to reflect the position that clients
must not be deprived, without some form of due process, of goods
and/or privileges that are rightfully theirs; furthermore, clients must
not be given low-salaried or unpaid work assignments that benefit the
institution but bear no clear relation to the client's rehabilitation
(Wexler, 1973). The studies examined subsequently are evaluated in
light of the above considerations.

CONCEPTUAL AND METHODOLOGICAL CRITIQUE
OF STUDIES

In general, the studies in our sample verified that certain techniques do improve specific behaviors in rehabilitation programs. The
programs described have emphasized self-care, improved work and
school performance, and the elimination of aggressive outbursts.
While it is true that those behaviors contribute to eventual rehabilitation, they are largely geared toward adjustment within the institutional
setting rather than toward independent adjustment to the outside world.
(Only the studies by Hunt and Azrin [1973] and by Haring and Mithaug
[1970] make adequate use of natural reinforcers in the community and
demonstrate programmed transition back to the "real" world.) Since
adequate transitional programs are notably lacking, the potential for
recidivism is very strong. We feel that the effectiveness of a behavioral approach to rehabilitation cannot be adequately tested unless
both institutional and transitional programs are combined into a single
project.

---

[*]A notable exception is the program at the Huntsville-Madison
Mental Health Center (Rinn et al., unpublished) in which discharged
patients are visited on a random basis, have their urine tested to
determine whether or not they are taking their medication, and receive
token reinforcement if the test is positive.

The methodology employed in the studies of positive reinforcement made no use of control groups, relying instead upon contingency reversals and multiple baselines. Although that alternate approach is appropriate for evaluating specific behavior-modification techniques, the evaluation of comprehensive rehabilitation programs requires more traditional control-group designs. Those studies in our sample group that chose not to use control groups also used no intragroup controls. Their major contribution, therefore, is in the evaluation of specific techniques rather than of comprehensive programs. The future may see a departure from that pattern, since several controlled studies of program evaluation are in progress, according to the reports we reviewed.

It should be noted that all the studies of positive reinforcement were introduced in institutions oriented toward custodial-care programs. Only the Draper project in Alabama (Rehabilitation Research Foundation, 1968, 1971, 1973a, 1973b) adequately separated the effects of the token reinforcement program from those of the enriched rehabilitation program; their preliminary data suggest that only the combined program is more effective than the traditional prison program. We look forward eagerly to learning the final results when this project is completed, and we suggest that such comprehensive studies be undertaken with other populations.

SUMMARY OF STUDIES

Studies of Positive Reinforcement

The most comprehensive study of positive reinforcement, the Draper Project, took place in the context of a comprehensive rehabilitation program in the Alabama state prison system. The project included an educational program, job training and relevant job placements in the institution, and vocational and behavioral counseling. It utilized a variety of reinforcers that were generally unavailable to inmates outside the program: permission to write extra letters, to go fishing, to visit a women's prison, to make a telephone call to someone outside the institution, to receive a copy of _Playboy_, to rent a television set, and so on. Good performance in the rehabilitation program also resulted in letters of recommendation to the parole board. The target behaviors incorporated specific performance criteria in the training and work programs, as well as personal self-care and care of individual living quarters.

The study of the Draper project includes a description of its sophisticated experimental design, which analyzes and compares the results of the token economy program and the training program in the absence of any concerted rehabilitation training effort. Although the final results of the study were not available when our review was conducted, preliminary data suggest that the entire rehabilitation package has been effective in increasing the number of hours worked, the amount of money earned, and the percentage of clients working during the first year after release from the institution. A number of other minor studies at Draper indicate that the token economy program was effective in changing institutional behavior—e.g., in increasing the rate of work of clients in the educational program. Careful analyses were also made of clients' needs prior to discharge, problems of post-discharge job placement, characteristics of persons who would later be recidivists, educational methods that are most effective with those clients, and techniques for and problems in the training of staff.

An interesting substudy compared the token-reinforcement system with the punitive-control methods that are ordinarily used in penal institutions. When authorities within the institution but outside the project demanded that inmates be punished for failure to care for their living quarters—e.g., make their beds—a marked improvement in bed-making behaviors occurred, but almost all other behaviors deteriorated—e.g., men stopped volunteering for assignments, number of fights increased, and so on. No such negative side-effects occurred when positive reinforcement was applied.

Although all the evaluation data on the Draper project are not yet available, we can comment on the project's shortcomings. Intermediate steps—job-placement services, transitional employment in outside settings, and halfway houses—may be needed to socialize inmates adequately to the outside world. A program that made such provisions for transition would undoubtedly be more effective than even the best rehabilitation program that is strictly limited to the confines of the prison walls.

Achievement Place (Wolf et al., 1971), a similarly comprehensive program for youthful offenders, indicates that token reinforcement is effective in modifying a variety of social, academic, self-care, prevocational, and family-living behavior problems. Its excellent methodology employs multiple baseline, baseline, and contingency reversals, but it does not use control groups. The project has produced a mine of information on behavioral-rating techniques, teaching methods, and methods of client self-government. Although the authors note anecdotally that the boys in their program seem to be progressing better than boys at the regular institution, they have not undertaken any systematic documentation of their observation. The Hawthorne

effect, which occurs when behavior changes due to the clients' awareness of his being observed and not as a result of treatment, could not
possibly explain the specific behavioral improvements, but it might
indeed contribute to the measured overall effectiveness of the programs.
Although no provision for transitional facilities are discussed, the
Achievement Place program manages to achieve quite a degree of
naturalness without them.

A report by Haring and Mithaug (1970) describes a demonstration
program in which a token system is used for adolescent school dropouts. The teenagers in the project build much of their own instructional
equipment, use automated programmed instructional devices, and are
gradually phased back into school. In several instances students are
made to compete with one another; in that population, contrary to general experience with academic failures, increased competition led to
improved academic performance. Almost all the boys in the program
remained involved in academic activities for at least a year, and
several returned to school full-time. However, the poor research
methodology precludes any final conclusions about that finding. Since
there is no control group, there is no way of evaluating the relative
effectiveness of the program as compared to other special education
programs.

An innovative study of a token-reinforcement program for aged
residents of a VA domiciliary at Wood, Wisconsin, was reported on
by Filer and O'Connell (1964). Project residents were variously rewarded with money, better living quarters, membership in an exclusive
club, increased privileges, and eligibility to participate in a self-
government program. The behaviors that were rewarded included
self-management, satisfactory management of medications and their
living quarters, and participation in some form of constructive work.
It was found that residents in the positive reinforcement program
became more active and less apathetic than subjects in a control
program. It was also shown that aged residents were much more
capable of independent and active behavior than had been previously
thought possible at this institution.

Several methodological problems plague that study. For example,
although control subjects were moved into a new ward that was physically identical to the experimental ward, they apparently were
deprived of the goods and privileges with which the experimental subjects were rewarded. In other words, the rewards may have been
"activating" for the residents, even if they had been given noncontin-
gently; thus, the system of reward for improved behavior was not
adequately tested. Obviously, a condition of noncontingent rewards is
a necessary control in such a study; without it there can be no adequate
test of the reward system.

Steffy's report (1971) on the Lakeshore Psychiatric Hospital, Toronto, Ontario, describes a reinforcement program for regressed mental patients. Its specific focus was on bedtime and mealtime behaviors and on controlling aggressive behaviors among regressed female psychiatric patients. Although it did improve mealtime and bedtime behaviors generally, such progress entailed the withholding of food from patients when their behavior was not appropriate. The project also failed to make use of more imaginative reinforcers within and outside the institution. Its recourse to deprivation raises ethical questions that prompt us to recommend against the replication of that program.

To control aggressive behavior, Lakeshore used a system of individualized behavioral-contingency contracts. That approach was found to be effective among patients whose aggressiveness was direct and overt. For the more withdrawn and manipulative patients, a more subtle analysis and a manipulation of communication contingencies were required. Since no control group was used, a Hawthorne effect is possible; but the exact timing of certain behavioral improvements coincides with treatment, thereby suggesting a cause-and-effect relationship. An interesting finding is that as their overt behavior improved, patients became more physiologically reactive. Like its counterparts, the study made no provisions for a gradual transitional phase-out between the hospital program and the outside world.

A study by Hunt and Zimmerman (1972) at New Castle State Hospital focused on patients with neurological disorders; some of them were retarded, and all had histories of severe seizure activity. Token reinforcement was effective in improving self-care and productivity in the setting of a sheltered workshop. The authors noted, however, that the teaching of specific job skills could be done more effectively by employers in the outside community than by a sheltered workshop in the hospital. Again, there is no mention of transitional programs.

The modification techniques employed in the New Castle program, including reversals of contingencies and gradually increased demands, were accompanied by gradually improved performance. Even without a control group, the methodology does tend to validate the effectiveness of the program, although it does not entirely isolate the expectancy effect.

In their study of Anna State Hospital's sophisticated community behavioral-treatment program for alcoholics, Hunt and Azrin (1973) found that patients in the behavioral program drank less, were more fully employed, and were institutionalized less frequently than control subjects, who received the standard hospital treatment program. The program was really not a token system at all, since it used only natural reinforcement—i.e., patients were taught, through behavioral

counseling, how to take advantage of the rewards offered by the real
world. The dramatic results strengthen our heuristic assumption that
the use of <u>natural reinforcement in the natural environment</u> should be
the treatment of choice with most groups. A Hawthorne effect is a
definite possibility here, however.

Studies of Goal Planning

Houts and Scott (1973) describe several studies of mental patients
in different kinds of environments using a goal-setting technique. In
each study, short-term and long-term goals are set with each patient,
according to the following criteria: involving the patient, setting
reasonable objectives, describing the patient's behavior when the goal
is reached, setting a deadline, and spelling out the method. Subjects
in the experimental group have their institutional programs specifically
oriented toward meeting their individual goals. Control subjects (and
the staff working with them) may work on their goals if they wish, but
their institutional programs remain unchanged. The experimental
subjects experienced much greater success in attaining their goals
than the control subjects. Despite the possible existence of a Hawthorne
effect among the experimental subjects and the lack of any systematic
investigation of the contribution of goal setting to the ultimate rehabilitation of patients, the approach has a good theoretical grounding both
in behavior modification and in McClelland's approach (McClelland and
Winter, 1969) of "need-achievement" training. It should be investigated
more thoroughly as a way of individualizing rehabilitation programs.

Studies of Programmed Instruction

A detailed study by H. D. B. Fredericks (1969) compared the
effect of the Doman Delacato Method with that of programmed instruction upon various kinds of muscle-coordination tasks. His outcome
criterion was a test of gross motor coordination. He found that while
the programmed techniques were more effective than no instructions
at all, the Doman Delacato Method was not.

Heber, Long, and Flanigan (1967) studied the relative effectiveness of traditional techniques for teaching braille and a special programmed method utilizing teaching machines. The differences between
groups were not dramatic: Subjects in the programmed-instruction
group were able to read 26-words-per-minute faster than subjects in
the control group after the study. There is some question whether

such minimal improvement warrants the investment in specialized
machinery.

RECOMMENDATIONS

The greatest contribution of the behavioral approach, as evidenced
by these studies, has been the creation of new techniques for managing
specific behaviors. Similarly, the strongest methodological aspects
of the studies are in evaluating the effects of specific techniques. Although the parameters of positive reinforcement and punishment have
been rather well documented, there is still room for further study.

Since the mechanics—i.e., specific rewards or punishments,
the types of target behaviors, and the particular contingencies used—
necessarily vary from setting to setting, there should be a reevaluation
in each setting that is substantially different.

The application of reinforcement and punishment contingencies
in community-based programs is an especially ripe area for further
study. Future researchers could focus on aftercare programs for
delinquents and the mentally disturbed (as in several reports not sur-
veyed here: Krop et al., 1972; Leberman et al., 1972; Fairweather
et al., 1969), primary prevention programs in schools and community
centers, job-training programs for the underprivileged, and outpatient-
treatment programs for a variety of chronic disorders.

It would also be interesting to compare clients in comprehensive
rehabilitation programs based on behavioral principles with those in
programs utilizing other methods or in those with persons not receiving
any rehabilitation services. The last type of studies would require
more rigorous use of control groups, follow-ups, and representative
sampling procedures than was the case for the studies we have
reviewed.

REFERENCES

Those reports with an asterisk were included in our sample of
477 projects. A complete list of all reports reviewed by the author is
available through the Disability and Health Economics Research Section, Rutgers University.

Atthowe, J. M., Jr., "Token Economies Come of Age." Behavior
    Therapy 4 (1973): 646-54.

Atthowe, J. M., Jr., and Krasner, L. "A Preliminary Report on
  the Application of Contingent Reinforcement Procedures (Token
  Economy on a 'Chronic' Psychiatric Ward)." Journal of Abnormal
  Psychology 73 (1968): 37–43.

Ayllon, T., and Azrin, N. H. The Token Economy: A Motivational
  System for Therapy and Rehabilitation. New York: Appleton,
  Century-Crofts, 1968.

Baer, D. M. "Some Remedial Uses of the Reinforcement Contingency."
  Research in Psychotherapy 3 (1968): 3–22.

Fairweather, G. W., Sanders, D. H., Cressler, D. L., and May-
  nard, H. Community Life for the Mentally Ill. Chicago: Aldine,
  1969.

*Filer, R. N., and O'Connell, D. D. "Motivation of Aging Persons."
  Journal of Gerontology 19 (1964): 15–22.

*Fredericks, H. D. B. A Comparison of the Doman-Delacato Method
  and Behavior Modification Method upon the Coordination of
  Mongoloids. Monmouth, Ore.: Teaching research, Oregon
  State System of Higher Education, 1969.

*Haring, N. G., and Mithaug, D. E. Final Report, VRA Grant No.
  RD-2794-P-69, An Investigation of Instructional Procedures
  for Increasing Performance Levels and Future Employment
  Opportunities of Marginal Students. Washington, D.C.: Social
  and Rehabilitation Service, 1970.

*Heber, R., Long, R., and Flanigan, P. A Study of Programmed
  Instruction in Braille. Madison: University of Wisconsin
  and Jonesville: Wisconsin School for the Visually Handicapped,
  1967.

*Houts, P. S., and Scott, R. A. Final Report: To Evaluate the
  Effectiveness of Achievement Motivation Training for Mental
  Patients Being Rehabilitated to the Community. Hershey:
  Pennsylvania State University, College of Medicine, 1973.

*Hunt, G. M., and Azrin, N. H. "A Community Reinforcement
  Approach to Alcoholism." Behavior Research and Therapy 11
  (1973): 91–104.

*Hunt, J. G. , and Zimmerman, J. Final Summary Report: Hospital
    Improvement Grant No. 51-P-70028-5-05m, Self-Care: Devel-
    opment and Vocational Rehabilitation. Washington, D. C.:
    NIMH, Public Health Service, 1972.

Krop, H. , Chudnovsky, N. , and Van Den Abell, T. "A Multilevel
    Behavioral Treatment Approach on Psychiatric Patients—No
    Tokens Please." Unpublished paper, VA Hospital, Gainesville,
    Fla. , 1972.

Leberman, R. P. , King, L. W. , and De Risi, W. "Building a Be-
    havioral Bridge to Span Continuity of Care." Unpublished paper,
    BAM Project and Clinical Research Units, Camarillo Neuro-
    psychiatric Institute, Camarillo, Calif. , 1972.

McClelland, D. C. , and Winter, D. G. Motivating Economic Achieve-
    ment. New York: Free Press, 1969.

*Rehabilitation Research Foundation. The Draper E and D Project:
    An Experimental Manpower Project for Training and Placement
    of Youthful Inmates of Draper Correctional Center at Elmore,
    Alabama, final report to the U.S. Department of Labor, Man-
    power Administration. Washington, D. C.: Government Printing
    Office, 1968.

____. Phase II Final Report, Experimental Manpower Laboratory for
    Corrections. Washington, D. C.: U. S. Department of Labor,
    Manpower Administration, 1971.

____. Phase III Final Report, Experimental Manpower Laboratory for
    Corrections. Washington, D. C.: U. S. Department of Labor,
    Manpower Administration, 1973a.

____. Phase IV Progress Report, Experimental Manpower Laboratory
    for Corrections. Washington, D. C.: U. S. Department of Labor,
    Manpower Administration, 1973b.

Rinn, R. C. , Tapp, L. , and Petrella, R. "The Use of Behavior
    Modification with Outpatients in a Community Mental Health
    Center." Unpublished paper, Huntsville-Madison County Mental
    Health Center, Huntsville, Ala. , n. d.

Sidman, M. The Tactics of Scientific Research. New York: Basic
    Books, 1960.

*Steffy, R. A. An Application of Learning Techniques to the Manage-
     ment and Rehabilitation of Severely Regressed, Chronically Ill
     Patients. Ottawa, Canada: Ontario Mental Health Foundation,
     1971.

Wexler, D. "Token and Taboo: Behavior Modification, Token Econ-
     omies, and the Law." California Law Review 61, no. 1, January
     1973, pp. 81-109.

Winnette, R. A., and Winkler, R. C. "Current Behavior Modification
     in the Classroom: Be Still, Be Quiet, Be Docile." Journal of
     Applied Behavior Analysis 5 (1972): 499-504.

*Wolf, M. M., Phillips, E. L., and Fixsen, D. L. Achievement
     Place: Behavior Modification with Predelinquents. Washington,
     D.C.: NIMH, Center for Studies of Crime and Delinquency,
     1971.

Adolescence is a time of increased conflicts and adjustment problems, even in normal populations. That emotional turbulence often dictates that techniques for treating and rehabilitating adolescents differ from those for adults or children. The unique physical and cognitive changes occurring during adolescence may add another dimension to the treatment of handicaps. This chapter will review studies done primarily with adolescent samples or populations in order to examine the roles of adolescence in general programs of treatment and rehabilitation.

In addition to having an awareness that adolescence compounds the problems inherent in treating certain handicaps, one must understand the relationship between adolescent conflicts and the specific handicaps involved. For example, physical and mental handicaps may become more significant as the adolescent matures: Cognitive deficiencies may seem more pronounced as a child grows toward physical adulthood. Likewise, physical or social handicaps may produce greater problems as the individual develops both psychologically and cognitively.

The types of handicaps to be covered in this chapter fall roughly into four groups: those of the mentally retarded, of the mentally ill and/or emotionally disturbed, of public offenders, and of delinquents, and socially and culturally disadvantaged. The four groups are not entirely distinct but overlap considerably, especially in the last three

---

This chapter was written by Peter Sheras, Intern in Clinical Psychology, Veterans Administration Hospital, Palo Alto, Calif.

categories; the relationship between mental illness, emotional disturbance, delinquency, and social disadvantage is in many cases interactive or causal. Any treatment of adolescents must be based on an understanding of that relationship, even though to date it may not be very well explicated by research and theory.

The type of study covered in this chapter would be of special interest to practitioners and administrators in both complete institutions and community-based programs. Although almost anyone involved in the treatment of adolescents can benefit from the information gathered in the type of research covered here, theoreticians have perhaps the least to gain, since most of the studies examined deal with the evaluation of the outcomes produced in specific programs. However, some theoretical inferences can be drawn from those cases where methods of treatment are compared with one another, as opposed to merely being compared with controls receiving no treatment. For the most part, however, the emphasis in these studies is placed upon treatment practices employed in programs of physical, mental, or social rehabilitation.

A total of 15 reports are considered in this chapter. Since, as we indicated above, the four content categories are not entirely distinct, some studies fall into more than one group. The breakdown is as follows: Five reports are in some way concerned with mental retardation; four deal with mental and/or emotional illness; six deal with public offenders; three discuss the socially and/or culturally disadvantaged.

INTERNAL VALIDITY AND METHODOLOGY

By and large, the collection of reports presents a picture of poor methodology and a lack of internal validity. Although a few reports are acceptable by almost any criteria of experimental design and methodology, most show either a lack of concern or competence with respect to design. The following discussion touches upon those aspects of the checklist that bear most significantly upon internal validity.

Sampling is, perhaps, the major detractor from internal validity in this set of studies. Very few were sampled well enough for their results to be generalizable to a larger population. Most samples were not representative—a shortcoming that is often attributable to the rigor of the screening criteria (e.g., many poorly motivated subjects may have been eliminated from the sample on the basis of the screening review). (For a fuller discussion of problems due to screening criteria, see the relevant part of the checklist review in Chapter 1.)

Since about half of the reports are either demonstrations or broad exploratory studies, they do not use experimental designs. However, five studies do use the separate control groups and the pretest/posttest design or some variant thereof.

In general, the statistical treatments in the group of reports are poor. Nonparametric statistics (usually percentage data or chi square) are used in nearly all the reports. Unfortunately, since the percentage data are often the sole "analysis" used, we can have just a vague picture of the results. In only one-third of the cases are statistics as sophisticated as that of a t-test, and multidimensional analysis is found only once. While it is true that design considerations in some cases do not warrant more elaborate statistical treatments, in other cases, more sophisticated statistics might have made better use of much of the available data.

Hypotheses, which clearly should be at the heart of any research project, are often poorly presented or totally lacking. Of the 15 reports in question, only 9 (or 60 percent) presented clearly testable hypotheses. In most of the other cases, the hypotheses were too vague to be tested or were nonexistent. Perhaps even more damaging testimony is that when hypotheses were presented in a testable way, in only two cases were alternative explanations discussed; a few others merely speculated about alternative explanations or hypotheses.

The control of external factors presented still another problem in many of the studies. Because control was frequently not discussed, it is difficult to know whether external factors were considered at all. Only two studies really attempted control of external factors. Five controlled, or attempted to control, internal environmental factors but gave no indication of their success in the effort. Those factors, internal or external, are of great importance, since they may interfere with the causal link between treatment and outcome variables. For example, a lack of concern with work environment may weaken the conclusions drawn about a program of psychiatric counseling designed to alter job-related attitudes and employment success.

As a group, the studies suffered from poor methodology; that was sometimes due to lack of hypotheses but was more often due to the nature of the population. Many of the studies had sampling problems because they were done with limited populations or in institutions that themselves were not representative of the population being studied. However, some of the errors—i.e., those not randomizing the sampling—are inexcusable. The quality of all but three of the reports in terms of internal validity ranged from fair to poor to very poor.

There seemed to be no one type of study, population, or setting that produced better research than any other. The quality of research seems to be a function of the individual researchers or of the idiosyncrasies of a given project. Judging from the group of studies at hand, with the exception of a few that are methodologically sound and well-controlled, the art of evaluation in the area would not appear to be very advanced. It is true that some populations are more difficult to study in a systematic way—e.g., adolescents dropping into a crash pad in Greenwich Village (Berkowitz et al., 1970). Nevertheless, many of the studies could have been based on much sounder evaluation techniques. Had the 14 out of 15 cases that were evaluated by in-house personnel been reviewed instead by an outside specialist conversant with the best methodologies and techniques, the findings might have been far more substantial. (For further discussion of this matter, see the overall analysis of the data in Chapter 14.)

To the extent that the methods tested in the studies are effective, the research has significant implications for policy choices in rehabilitation. Although the studies represent a conglomeration of techniques used on different handicaps, as a whole they tend to show that specific improvements can be made in preparing the adolescent for the world of work. Some studies are so poor methodologically that little or no inference about policy utility can be made. However, in many cases, interesting and innovative techniques demand our attention, even though the evaluation of those techniques does not unequivocally support their validity.

Basically, the reports present two treatment models. The first submits the handicapped adolescent to a specific therapeutic technique and then measures the results in terms of adjustment. That model, used in a number of reports, is exemplified by the socially disadvantaged youths' experience in survival camping in the wilderness followed by the measurement of behavioral changes upon their return (Collingwood). Another study compares two therapy techniques: behavior modification and transactional analysis (Jesness, 1972). Although the specific policy utility of each of these studies appears to be sizable, the techniques are actually applicable to very limited situations, populations and/or environments. The second model reflects the coordination of services in a comprehensive multitreatment program for the handicapped adolescent. (For a more detailed analysis of coordination of services see Chapter 12.) For each handicap, a different array of services is coordinated. The major thrust is to provide for the rehabilitation of the client from an institution or sheltered environment into a real-life circumstance, by coordinating "inside" and "outside" services. Coordination may take the form of work orientation through jobs in outside industry, followed by counseling after job placement. Vocational skills can also be taught in sheltered workshops that allow the adolescent to increase his or her self-image regardless of the type of training. The second model, despite its lack of experimental support in the studies, has the strongest implications for rehabilitation practitioners.

One task of future research should be the replication with controls of programs whose evaluations were methodologically weak. The findings indicate that more longitudinal studies are necessary to confirm the staying power of the results. (It is disturbing to realize that of the reports cited in this chapter only two include follow-ups, while two others suggest a follow-up be undertaken.) One conclusion that does seem clear is the statement that the best direction to follow in the treatment of adolescents is toward a "comprehensive" approach.

The difficulties in estimating the magnitude of costs and benefits are compounded by the poor caliber of many of the studies. If it can be shown that extensive benefits can result from the coordination of existing services (e.g., jobs in the business sector with therapeutic orientation in institutions), then the costs may be comparatively small. However, if successful adolescent rehabilitation requires complete comprehensive programs, the costs may be greater. In other words, the relationship between cost and benefit varies from one situation to another. In cases where adolescents undergo comprehensive in-house treatment, the cost may be lower compared to situations where clients may come and go as they please, participating in programs as they see fit.

REVIEW OF KEY PROJECTS

Because this chapter is based upon a number of different types of reports, it is almost impossible to present an "average" or archetypical report. It may be instructive, however, to present a brief summary of three reports representing different areas of the domain involved. Those that have been selected are the best in terms of method and validity. The poor quality of many of the other reports has prompted us to exclude them from consideration, even as examples of less-than-mediocre research.

Slutzky, 1963

The study intended to provide and evaluate the outcomes of a vocational rehabilitation program for emotionally disturbed adolescents from 16 to 21 years of age.

It chose 77 subjects who had WAIS Full Scales IQ of 75 or above and who were capable of working and interested in doing so. The subjects were provided with mechanical- and clerical-training facilities. One goal of the program was to obtain positive group identification.

Applicants and their families were carefully screened and discussed
by the staff. After entering the program, the adolescent was evaluated
in a number of work settings with different work supervisors. When
enough progress was made, the adolescent was placed in an employment setting. After one month on the job he was automatically terminated from the program. At the beginning and end of the training
program the client was administered an employment-readiness and a
psychiatric scale. Of the 50 percent of the experimental group who
were employed, 55 percent were still employed after six months.
Data analyzed from the scales showed that the rehabilitation group
had more favorable scores initially and more improvement than the
control group. They also received scores showing greater ego
strength.

Although the sampling procedure makes the results a bit suspect
(only the motivated subjects were chosen to begin with), the results
do seem positive and useful.

Jesness, 1972

This study compared the effectiveness of two treatment methods—
behavior modification and transactional analysis—in rehabilitating
institutionalized delinquents. Two nearly identical institutions were
chosen, with approximately 400 boys in each. Boys entering the
system were randomly assigned to one of the two centers, each using
a different treatment program. The dependent variables were parole
rates, institutional progress, inmate/staff attitudes, and social
climate. After 18 months, results indicated a) less recidivism on
parole among subjects from both experimental groups; b) marked
positive effect on social climate in both groups; c) transactional analysis subjects rated small groups as more helpful, while behavior modification group rated education program highest; d) more mature
subjects participated actively in both programs. The last was expected
in the TA program but unanticipated in the BM program.

This study provides some empirical facts about treatment
outcomes. It would appear to have great policy utility and also provides for a theoretical discussion of the reasons for the particular
outcome.

Collingwood

The extent of the project was to develop and implement a chal-
lenging survival camping program as a means of rehabilitating

culturally and socially disadvantaged youth. It was designed to make
use of the therapeutic potential within the process of camping and
attempting to survive against nature with others. Subjects were 20 boys
from training schools, Rehabilitation Service First Offender Project
and a large rehabilitation facility. There were eight controls. Treatment variables included physical training in camping skills, backpack-
ing, group counseling, and recreation. Dependent measures were
physical fitness, self-concept, and behavior. Following the three-
week program, participants showed a) decreased heart rates (physical
fitness); b) significant increase in self-concept ratings; c) significant
increase in internal control; d) increased positive behavior and
decreased negative behavior as rated by parent and counselor.

Although clearly not applicable to a wide range of populations,
this report provides a concise picture of a specific technique and a
reasonable judgment of its success. The policy utility and benefits
are readily apparent.

RECOMMENDATIONS

It is difficult to make a general statement about the implementation of the research findings reviewed in this chapter. Suffice it to
say that their implementation should be based on additional research
to validate them. Although specific studies may be instructive, they
point most notably to the need for further quality research.

The need for further research is evident both from the poor
quality of the reports included herein and from the dearth of resources
on such a large population (adolescents account for about 20 percent
of the current U.S. population). Many of the reports are, by their
own admission, not experiments but uncontrolled demonstrations. It
is the lack of control that makes the conclusions so difficult to generalize. We feel that competent researchers need to work hand in hand
with clinicians and administrators to develop more valid evaluation
mechanisms for adolescent-rehabilitation programs. Research on
adolescents is especially necessary, because the life phase itself is
still so poorly understood from an etiological standpoint as well as
from a developmental and a clinical one.

We feel that those who administer programs are too involved
with them to do an adequate scientific evaluation. When confronted
with a limited budget and a choice between spending money for research
or service expansion, practitioners generally opt for the latter. To
fill the resulting research gap, the grantor can either provide a larger
budget or require a more serious research commitment.

There exists a great potential and need for valid research with handicapped adolescents. Adequate treatment of adolescents can obviously have an impact upon the later need for adult rehabilitation, especially in terms of mental and cultural deficiencies. Good research with adequate follow-up is, therefore, a most pressing concern.

REFERENCES

The reports in this section are those which the author used in preparing the chapter. Although all the reports below are in our sample, the author has not been responsible for the rating of any reports.

Berkowitz, L., Meltzer, R., Zicht, L., et al. Pilot and Research Project for Dissident Youth—("Hippies")—in East Village of New York City. New York: The Educational Alliance. February 1970.

Collingwood, T. R. Survival Camping: A Therapeutic Mode for Rehabilitating Problem Youth. Fayetteville, Ark.: Arkansas Rehabilitation and Research Training Center.

De Haven, G. E., Bruce, J. D., and Bryan, D. C. Remediation of Coordination Deficits in Youth with Minimal Cerebral Dysfunction. Devon, Pa.: The Devereux Foundation Institute for Research and Training, 1971.

Fahey, F. J., Banks, R. R., and Kiekbusch, R. Assisting Youth Toward Socio-Economic Adjustment. Notre Dame, Ind.: University of Notre Dame, 1967.

Geteles, F., Bierman, A., Gaza, C., Kelley, E., and Rusalem, H. A Cooperative Vocational Pattern for In-School Mentally Retarded Youth. Orange, N.J.: Occupational Center of Essex County, 1967.

Hazian, D. J. Preventive Rehabilitation—A Promise for the Future. Providence, R.I.: State Division of Vocational Rehabilitation, 1968.

Jesness, C. Differential Treatment of Delinquents in Institutions. Sacramento, Calif.: Department of Youth Authority, 1972.

Lane, J. P. Omaha Public Schools Work Experience Program.
     Omaha, Neb.: Department of Special Services, 1968.

Lauderdale, M., Haskins, J. R., and Kott, R. L. Rehabilitation of
     Intractable Defective Delinquents. Mexia, Tex.: Mexia State
     School, 1972.

Orzack, L. H., Cassell, J. T., and Halliday, H. Experiences of
     Former Special Class Students and an Educational Work/Experi-
     ence Program for Secondary School Educable Mentally Retarded
     Students, Parents and Friends of Mentally Retarded Children of
     Bridgeport, Inc. Bridgeport, Conn.: Bridgeport, Inc., 1969.

Root, A., Benney, C., and Small, L. A Demonstration in Rehabili-
     tation of the Mentally Ill Adolescent and Young Adult. New York:
     Altro Health and Rehabilitation Services, 1966.

Slutzky, J. E. "A Structured Therapeutic Work-Study Program for
     Emotionally Disturbed Adolescents." Unpublished final report,
     Berman School, Inc., Freeport, N.Y., 1963.

Stephenson, R. M., Scarpitti, F. R., The Rehabilitation of Delinquent
     Boys. New Brunswick, N.J.: Rutgers, the State University,
     1967.

West, J. A., Keith, D. L., and Vialle, H. "Vocational Rehabilitation
     in Juvenile Delinquency—A Planning Program." Unpublished
     final report, Division of the State Board for Vocational Educa-
     tion, Oklahoma City, Okla., 1964.

Zivan, M. "Youth in Trouble. A Vocational Approach." Unpublished
     final report, the Children's Village, Dobbs Ferry, N.Y., 1966.

**REHABILITATION
AND PUBLIC OFFENDERS**

After a brief preliminary examination of 65 studies dealing primarily with rehabilitation involving a social-work component of public offenders, we shall discuss more fully those projects in correctional rehabilitation. The former were included so as to keep the social-work chapter from becoming unmanageable; the latter were included as the area of special consideration for this chapter.

The studies were categorized by handicaps. Of the total 65 projects, the largest proportion of reports dealt with mental illness, alcoholism, mental retardation, and crime and delinquency. However, the single largest category, representing approximately 30 percent of the studies, was that which dealt explicitly with criminal and delinquent offenders.

Many of the reports could not really be considered as basic research efforts; rather, they tended to be final reports relating to demonstration projects, and as such, merely stated the rehabilitative strategy employed and the number of clients served over a given period of time. Undoubtedly, the simple reporting mechanisms developed for the projects could have been utilized as part of an ongoing evaluative research effort.

Another shortcoming arose from the practice of many projects attempting to measure "success" in terms of clients' program completion and/or the project's ability to secure immediate job placement.

This chapter was written by Joanne Jankovic, student, Graduate School of Social Work, Rutgers University; Project Specialist at Bureau of Research Planning and Program Development of the New Jersey Division of Youth and Family Services.

Client follow-up was rare and there was no attempt to follow up individuals who were rejected for services.

Table 7.1, which shows the distribution of reports by type of research design and handicap, indicates that 55 percent did not utilize any type of experimental design. The pattern may be due to the difficulties inherent in conducting scientific research within a human-service program; the structure of such programs does not allow for strong control, such as, for example, the comparison of informal client screening versus random selection.

That correctional-rehabilitation programs made more extensive use of experimental designs can be attributed to several factors. Since most of their client population was drawn from institutions, they had built-in means of control—e.g., ability to make random assignment to different treatment milieus, training programs, and so forth. Also, pretest data are readily obtainable through utilization of case records, evaluations, psychological tests, previous offenses, and so on. Finally, follow-up data are available through existing reporting mechanisms—parole violations and rearrest rates—that provide a consistent means of tracking ex-client activities. All of those special characteristics of the correctional setting combine to provide an adequate groundwork for quality research.

REHABILITATION AND CORRECTIONS

In recent years correctional programs have begun to shift away from punishment and towards treatment and rehabilitation. The past two decades have seen the increased utilization of casework, therapy, educational services, and medical services within the criminal justice system. The introduction of educational and treatment programs was intended as much to humanize the system as it was to humanize the offender.

Only within the last few years has there been a significant effort to measure the effectiveness of various correctional programs—i.e., the effect of an inmate's exposure to certain treatment variables upon his readjustment to community life. Such evaluative research has consisted largely of follow-up studies attempting to relate various treatments to postrelease adjustment. All evaluative studies have been beset by the difficulty arising from the lack of empirical scales regarding "success," total/partial rehabilitation, and failure. Recidivism data over time appear to be inadequate for the task.

Some of the studies reviewed represent the most extensive research that has been conducted in the juvenile and adult correctional field over the past several years—most notably, studies from the

TABLE 7.1

Reports on Rehabilitation and Public Offenders, by Type of Design and Handicap

Handicap	One-Shot Case	One Group Pretest/ Posttest	Static Group	Pretest/ Posttest Control Group	Posttest Only Control Group	Equivalent Time Series	Nonequivalent Control Group	Multiple Time Series	Other	None	Total
Visual impairment	—	—	—	—	1	—	—	—	—	1	2
Hearing impairment	—	—	—	—	—	—	1	—	—	—	1
Mental retardation	2	—	—	—	—	—	—	—	1	4	7
Mental illness	—	1	—	—	1	—	—	1	—	6	9
Alcoholism	—	—	—	1	—	—	—	—	—	3	4
Drug abuse	—	—	—	—	—	—	—	—	—	1	1
Public offenders	—	—	1	5	2	1	1	—	2	7	19
Educationally, socially disadvantaged	—	—	—	2	—	—	—	—	—	4	6
Other	1	—	—	1	3	—	—	—	1	8	14
Total	3	1	1	9	7	1	2	1	4	36	65

Source: Compiled by the authors.

74

California Youth Authority (Palmer, 1972; Jesness, 1971) and Department of Corrections (Spencer and Berecochea, 1971; Rudoff, 1969). (We were unable to include all of the studies done by these agencies.) Also included are a series of research/demonstration projects conducted within the federal correctional system. We were unable to obtain information from the Seattle part of this program, where much of the overall data analysis was to be done; our review may be lacking in this instance. Overall, the research was directed toward evaluating the effectiveness of the following types of programs:

- Court diversion projects (Zimring, 1973)
- Group homes—for youths—as alternatives to incarceration (Palmer, 1972)
- Intensive parole/probation projects (Collins, 1969; Stendebach and Adams, 1968)
- Institutional treatment milieus, utilizing differential treatment approaches (Rudoff, 1969; Seckel, Woodring, and Raab)
- Institutional vocational/academic programs, both for adult and youthful offenders (Coombs and Clemmons, 1965; Basinas et al., 1973)
- Postinstitutional vocational rehabilitation programs (Ericson and Moberg, 1967). (For a discussion of behavior modification techniques, see Chapter 5.)

Most of the studies employed experimental research designs, but there was considerable variation in the quality of research. Institutional-treatment projects and group home study represented the highest quality of research, while the vocational rehabilitation studies were

TABLE 7.2

Ratings of 19 Studies on Rehabilitation of Offenders,
by Type of Program Studied

Type of Program	Mean Research Methodology Rating	Mean Policy Utility Rating
Court diversion	7.5	7.5
Group homes	10.0	10.0
Parole/probation	5.0	5.3
Institutional/treatment	9.5	10.0
Institutional vocational training	5.4	6.0
Postinstitutional vocational training	5.5	6.1

generally of the poorest quality. The latter group consisted mainly of institutional vocational-training and educational programs. The repor in that area tended toward description rather than evaluation. The ratings of programs is shown in Table 7.2.

Internal Validity

Most of the projects reviewed studied samples of institutional and/or parole populations. Approximately half of the studies did not utilize adequate sampling procedures; since they relied on certain screening criteria—arrest/drug-use history, psychological test scores, and subjective case-records evaluations—to select program participants, their sample selection tended to be biased. Also, when comparison groups were used, insufficient information was given regarding their formation. The result of the above inadequacies was that even though large populations may have been studied, the question able sampling procedures cast doubts about the project's results.

The remainder of the studies did employ adequate sampling procedures. Six used random sampling and the random assignments of subjects to different treatment and control groups. And their samples were sufficiently large (200 to 1,300 subjects), representing the total institutional admissions and releases during a one- to three-year time period.

Approximately two-thirds of the correctional reports were experimental in nature. Of all the studies utilizing experimental designs, only one was preexperimental.* The research projects employing experimental designs also used sampling procedures (random sampling and assignments) that made for representative populations. In addition, the majority of the projects had developed testable hypotheses. Unfortunately, no project was able to control maximally for external factors; hence, it was difficult to discern whether observed behavioral changes resulted from exposure to particular treatment variable(s) or from exposure to other variables that the researcher was unable to control.

The major difficulty encountered by all the projects appears to be their inability to control those variables that were not a part of the immediate treatment. It is perhaps presumptuous to assume that a particular treatment program will significantly reduce recidivism

---

*Preexperimental designs are defined as those in which the researcher does not have control over randomization and scheduling of data collection.

rates, when that treatment is only one small element of the institution's
on-going operation. None of the studies attempted to assess either the
impact of institutional life on behavior (peer influence, staff-inmate
interaction patterns, and so forth), or the reception accorded to an
innovative treatment method by security and/or administrative staff.

Clearly, there is a need for some other means of measuring
outcome. Although treatment or vocational-training programs may
have some measurable impact (e.g., improved human relations or
work skills), they should not be evaluated primarily on the basis of
recidivism data. There is no consensus among the studies on a definition of the term "recidivism"; a person was variously considered a
recidivist if he were rearrested but not recommitted; if he violated
parole (violation may constitute acts that are not criminal offenses);
if he were rearrested and returned to the institution. (Careful note
should be made of the lack of consensus when recidivism rates are
reported.)

There is considerable need to study individuals who have successfully returned to community life. Especially useful would be a
determination of those factors related to positive readjustment—e.g.,
marital/family relationships, employability, peer group influence,
and so on.

Policy Utility

Overall, the studies produced little empirical evidence substantiating that one particular type of treatment was superior to another.
For example, in our sample there were no studies that compared the
effectiveness of institutional versus noninstitutional care. But the
research does yield some information regarding the effect of a particular type of treatment on different types of offenders; such data are
especially abundant in studies conducted by the California Youth
Authority (CYA), which utilized a behavioral classification system
(Interpersonal Maturity Levels) to match behavior with a particular
type of treatment. However, since most of that research has been
conducted under the auspices of one agency and since many of its
findings have been criticized (see Lerman, 1968; Warren and Palmer,
1966), more extensive research is obviously needed.

The effectiveness of vocational rehabilitation for public offenders,
both institutional and postinstitutional, is highly questionable. There
was no significant difference in parole performance between groups
exposed to experimental-treatment variables (group therapy, intensive
casework, prerelease vocational program) and groups exposed to
traditional methods (surveillance, control, menial tasks, and so on)—

all the studies of vocational rehabilitation programs showed similar
findings. One research project conducted at the California Institution
of Women (Spencer and Berecochea, 1971) studied the success of
paroled women in finding employment in the fields in which they were
trained while in the institution. It found that, after 12 months on
parole, only 32 percent of the women available for employment were
employed in fields related to their institutional training; a woman who
was trained in a particular field before her incarceration was more
likely to hold a job in that field after release. Those findings raised
a question as to whether vocational programs in prisons are actually
geared to preparing individuals with employable skills for entry into
the labor market or whether they merely meet narrow institutional
needs.

Research on the effectiveness of community-based treatments—
halfway houses, day treatment, and group homes, and so forth—is
just beginning to emerge. Available data have implications for the
entire correctional rehabilitation process, substantiating the growing
awareness that certain individuals do not have to be institutionalized
to be rehabilitated. Statistical analysis of experimental and control
group data from a New York study of a pilot court service project
(Zimring, 1973; Aronson et al., 1972) showed that early intervention
can divert offenders from further involvement in the criminal justice
system. And the use of community-based group homes for delinquents
is supported by evidence found in a study conducted by the California
Youth Authority (Palmer, 1972). But even though those programs
report some relative effectiveness and do represent considerable
potential in the treatment of delinquent and adult offenders, there
is still a pressing need for further research comparing their effectiveness with traditional treatment methods.

SPECIFIC PROJECTS

The two projects we have selected for further discussion,
California Group Home Project (Palmier 1972) and the Probational
Offenders Rehabilitation and Training (PORT) project of Rochester,
Minnesota (Tyce and Lindgren, 1972), should be of special interest
to those who are engaged in experimental correctional rehabilitation.
A review of their innovative treatment programs and of the difficulties
attendant upon attempts at systematic study of the effectiveness of
such projects should prove particularly useful.

The California Group Home Project, funded by NIMH, was an
effort to study the differential use of group homes within the California
Youth Authority Community Treatment Project (CTP). The develop-

ment of the project was influenced by earlier placement difficulties encountered within the CTP, which had concentrated on out-of-home placements as deterrents to future delinquent activites (30 percent of CTP's experimental subjects were in facilities other than the family environment). The study sample, consisting of youths committed by the courts to the state correctional system after an average of five arrests, was not representative of a typical probation caseload. Assignment of the youths to a group home facility was based upon the Interpersonal Maturity Levels classification system. The nine group home facilities studied during the project's duration were categorized into six types:

Type I: Protective. For immature and dependent children. It provides normal family living and is operated by a married couple who supervise for long periods of time.

Type II: Containment. For children who are culturally conforming delinquents. Main characteristics are firm, objective authority; demand for conforming, productive behavior.

Type III: Boarding. Home for more "mature and complex children who are in early stages of emancipation, but who do not have enough strength to be on their own." Main characteristics: serves as "base" for child while he resolves internal conflicts, identity problems, and so on; nonthreatening parents allow children the initiative in developing relationships.

Type IV: Temporary Community Care. Short-term placement when confinement or independent living is inappropriate. Also serves as interim for changes between placements.

Type V: Restriction. Home serves as substitute for detention. Placement is for ten days or fewer.

Type VI: Individualized Home. Long-term, "open-ended" placement resource for youths who would benefit from an environment providing family-like atmosphere and opportunity for positive adult relationships.

During three years of group home operation, 104 separate placements were made. Findings showed that youths in long-term placement performed little better than those who were not placed. Follow-up showed the following record of parole failure:

	Experimentals	Controls
15 months	17%	31%
24 months	33%	43%

The most successful group homes were boarding homes for higher-maturity youths and temporary care for all types. Containment homes were unsuccessful. Self-ratings and staff ratings indicate that there was moderate success in the selection of adequate group home operators.

The project isolates several programmatic difficulties encountered in attempting to establish the homes:

- Group home operator's inability to deal with a child's particular problem
- Number of referrals for Type V were below preproject expectations
- Difficulties in "matching" group home operators, parole agents, and youths

The above organizational problems hampered the development of new resources in that they impeded the assessment of external factors as they related to the implementation of an innovative service model. In terms of costs, the group homes serve as relatively economical resources, compared to more elaborate, highly professionalized treatment modalities.

The second project has significant implications for further research. The PORT project in Minnesota employed an innovative treatment strategy. Although it did not use a quality evaluative design, its basic data should especially be helpful to correctional rehabilitation people who are concerned about the costs of treatment and are interested in implementing intervention programs within the community.

Specifically, the PORT program is an effort to commit first offenders to a community halfway house instead of incarcerating them or placing them on probation. It serves individuals ranging from 14 to 47 years of age. Entrance into the program is voluntary, even though referral is made through the court. Participants provide their own funds to reside in the program, while volunteer residential counselors receive room and board for staying at the facility.

The living environment is based on a value system in which controls over behavior and freedom of movement can vary from the most restrictive confinement of activities to the most open and permissive atmosphere.

During the four years of its operation, the program has served 60 individuals; 19 cases of failure were reported in which individuals were committed to institutions. The average cost per resident is considerably below the costs in state correctional facilities. It is difficult to account specifically for the project's considerable degree of success; there is no sure way of knowing what role if any was played by early court-diversion efforts, the particular treatment approach used, the physical location of the project within a community, and the employment of nonprofessionals in the rehabilitation process.

CONCLUSIONS AND RECOMMENDATIONS

Overall, the studies regarding the rehabilitation of delinquent
and adult offenders exhibited somewhat better quality research than
the remainder of the sample reviewed. Further assessment of the
correctional rehabilitation studies failed to indicate outstanding
effectiveness of one program relative to another. Of the many difficulties encountered in employing experimental research, the most
notable was the lack of any attempt to control all variables impinging
upon the phenomena being studied.

The implications for further research in correctional rehabilitation are numerous. First, there is a basic need to determine the
types of institutional programs that are most effective. As mentioned
earlier, there is a need for additional criteria with which to measure
outcome and from which to determine the impact of particular institutional processes upon individual behavior. Second, studies relating
to the application of a particular treatment strategy must be based
upon a solid body of knowledge or theory. Third, there is a need for
further study of factors contributing to individual success—i.e.,
whether it results from some set of personal characteristics or from
exposure to certain treatment variables. And, finally, we need comparative data on the effectiveness of community-based versus institutional programs. As more and more states are turning to
community-based programs, the need and opportunity to pursue such
research becomes even more apparent.

REFERENCES

Those reports with an asterisk were included in our sample of
477 projects. A complete list of all reports reviewed by the author
is available through the Disability and Health Economics Research
Section of the Bureau of Economic Research at Rutgers University.

*Aronson, H., Olgiati, E. J., Friedman, D. H., and Rubinstein, D.
  Manhattan Court Employment Project, Phase II. New York:
  Vera Institute of Justice, 1972.
*Basinas, A. W., Stoddard, J. G., Ferstl, J. H., and Powers, S. B.
  Work-Release Study Program. Madison, Wis.: Wisconsin
  Division of Corrections, 1973.
*Collins, J. A. Springfield Federal Offender Rehabilitation Project.
  Springfield, Ill.: Illinois Division of Vocational Rehabilitation,
  1969.

*Coombs, K. A., and Clemmons, G. K. An Analysis of the Academic Educational Program in Washington State Adult Correctional Institutions. Olympia, Wash.: Department of Institutions, 1965.

*Ericson, R. C., and Moberg, D. O. The Rehabilitation of Parolees— The Application of Comprehensive Psycho-Social Vocational Services in the Rehabilitation of Parolees. Minneapolis, Minn.: Minneapolis Rehabilitation Center.

*Jesness, C. F. "The Preston Typology Study: An Experiment with Differential Treatment in an Institution," Journal of Research in Crime and Delinquency 8 (1971): 38-52.

Lerman, P. "Evaluating the Outcome of Institutions for Delinquents: Implications for Research and Social Policy." Social Work 13 (July 1968): 55-64.

*Palmer, T. Differential Placement of Delinquents in Group Homes. Sacramento, Calif.: California Department of Youth Authority, 1972.

*Rudoff, A. A Measure of Casework in Corrections. San Jose, Calif.: Center for Interdisciplinary Studies, San Jose State College, 1969.

*Seckel, J. P., Woodring, T. M., and Raab, B. J. Summary of Assessment of Vocational Rehabilitation Program at Preston School of Industry. Sacramento, Calif.: California Department of Youth Authority.

*Spencer, C., and Berecochea, J. E. Vocational Training at the California Institution for Women: An Evaluation. Sacramento, Calif.: Research Division, Department of Corrections, 1971.

*Stendebach, E. H., and Adams, I. R. Texas Federal Offenders Rehabilitation Project. Austin, Tex.: Division of Vocational Rehabilitation, Texas Education Agency, 1969.

Tyce, F. A., and Lindgren, J. G. Probationed Offenders Rehabilitation and Training. Rochester, Minn.: PORT of Olmsted County, 1972.

Warren, R., and Palmer, T. Evaluation of Community Treatment for Delinquents, Report No. 7. Sacramento, Calif.: California Youth Authority, 1966.

*Zimring, F. The Court Employment Project. New York: Court Employment Project, 1973.

8

REHABILITATION AND SPECIAL EDUCATION

Special education refers to educational provisions for those individuals who cannot achieve adequately within traditional general educational systems. It may include special teaching competencies, teaching procedures, types of instruction, devices, or school services. The services offered will vary depending on both type and degree of exceptionality, as well as on individual characteristics. Programs may range from a short period of time to many years. Traditional subgroups within special education are mental retardation, emotional disturbance, social maladjustment, hearing impairment, visual impairment, communication disorders, orthopedic handicaps, chronic medical problems, neurological impairment, perceptual impairment, specific learning disabilities, and (excluded from consideration in this project) superior cognitive abilities. Each area includes a broad range of ability or disability.

Reports were reviewed for the following groups: visual impairment, speech impairment, orthopedic handicaps, mental retardation, mental illness (including both emotionally disturbed and, to a lesser extent, socially maladjusted), and educationally disadvantaged (primarily cultural minority groups). The "other" classification includes populations with multiple handicaps and those for whom a primary classification could not be determined. Each category is considered

---

This chapter was written by Ivan Z. Holowinsky, Professor and Chairman, Department of Psychological Foundations, Rutgers University, and Ruth Ann Hebble, graduate student, Special Education Curriculum, Graduate School of Education, Rutgers University. A complete list of the 78 reports reviewed in this chapter is available through the Disability and Health Economics Research Section.

in a broad sense, since precise definitions may vary. Since multiple
handicaps are common, the category under consideration generally
represents the primary problem. Of the 78 project reports covered
in this chapter on special education, 37 were concerned with programs
for the mentally retarded. Other programs were for those with visual
impairments (N = 12), speech impairments (N = 5), hearing impairments (N = 6), and the mentally ill (N = 6).

Of the 77 projects that reported sufficient sampling information,
the sample sizes covered a wide range, with the largest percentage of
reports (32.5) being in the 101 to 250 range. For 60 (78.9 percent) of
the 78 reports, reviewers expressed doubts concerning the generalizability on the basis of sampling shortcomings; inadequate sample size
was not the major flaw: lack of representativeness and poor sampling
procedures were each noted in about one-fifth of the reports, and
some combination of those three types of problems was noted in 23
(29.5 percent) of the projects. A frequent sampling weakness stemmed
from the inclusion of all those who were referred or of all who survived a screening process. And samples were often so poorly defined
that it was impossible to determine what population was being represented.

Most projects employed some combination of two or more of the
data sources included on the checklist. Those projects using only a
single data source most often used tests given by researchers. Appropriateness of data sources was not included in the checklist.

One difficulty in gathering data was the handling of nonresponses,
refusals, and dropouts, with dropouts posing the most frequent problems. In more than half of the project reports where incomplete data
were noted, the handling of those data was unclear, and the effects
may have ranged from minimal to very significant. For example, of
51 projects that reported dropouts, three included them in the data
analysis, 21 specifically excluded them, and 27 merely described the
dropouts and did not specify how they were treated. In some projects,
reporting of the sample was sufficiently hazy to arouse suspicions
about the incompleteness of the data; in others incomplete data were
due to internal problems, such as differentially administered tests.

METHODOLOGY AND DATA ANALYSIS

The question, whether the research design was experimental,
was answered for 77 of the projects. Of these, 49 (63.6 percent) were
classified by reviewers as experimental designs while 28 (36.4 percent) were not. Nonexperimental designs were chiefly demonstration
projects or pilot studies. The one-shot case study (20 projects) was

the most frequent type of experimental design, followed by 11 one-group pretest/posttest designs. Control groups were involved in only 11 projects. It is true that the nature of the research we reviewed does not lend itself readily to designs involving control groups, yet many reports attributed changes to treatment with little or no control for developmental or spontaneous changes, thus limiting their credibility.

The projects varied widely in their consideration of variables that may be related to disability, but, taken as a group, the control of or analysis of the effects of such variables was poor. Age and type of disability were the only two variables analyzed or controlled for by more than half of the reports. Sex, intelligence, and severity of handicap were included as variables in slightly less than half of the projects. The remaining variables listed were either most often not considered or merely described for the sample and mentioned as possibly having an effect. For example, subject attitude, which may exert a powerful influence, was not considered in 79.5 percent of the 78 reports; it was merely described or cited as having a possible effect in an additional 5.1 percent of reports.

Control for external influences tended to be poor. Reviewers noted that only 17.1 percent of the reports used some type of control for external influences. There was no control in more than three-quarters of the projects. Internal project environments, however, did not seem to be a major cause of bias in results.

The treatment or independent variables employed covered a broad spectrum of areas, including treatments such as speech, physical therapy, counseling, medical treatment, and vocational training, as well as traditional special education programs.

The most frequently used dependent variable was employed/not employed, followed by success/failure and test ratings. A frequent problem was poor definition of dependent variables, especially where value judgments on the part of the project staff were involved—for example, in success/failure or improved/not improved. The time between end of treatment and measurement of effect was not clearly specified in almost half of the reports. A third problem was that the generally short time lapse between treatment and measurement of effects may not have been appropriate to some changes that were being measured, such as employed/not employed, where a long-term effect is desired.

A related problem was the general lack of follow-up. In almost 90 percent of the reports either there was no mention of follow-up or follow-up was merely suggested as a good idea.

In general, the statistics used were employed properly, but treatment of the data collected was limited to descriptive statistics in the majority of reports. A major problem was that many reports made

statements about significant changes, improvements, or differences
solely on the basis of an inspection of descriptive statistics and without having tested statistical significance. Evaluation of most of the
projects was conducted by project staff. Where such in-house evaluation was coupled with poorly defined dependent variables, the problem
was especially acute. In other words, many reports force one to rely
solely on the opinion of project staff as to the efficacy of projects.

POLICY UTILITY

From the preceding discussion, it should not be surprising that
research methodology ratings tended to be low: 61 reports (78.2 percent) were rated as low (one, two, or three); two reports were given
a rating of eight and the remainder fell into the four to seven range.
Criteria used in determining overall policy utility ratings
included current trends in the field of special education as well as
those factors included in the checklist. However, chiefly because of
poor research methodology, 80.8 percent of the projects were rated
as having low policy utility (ratings of one, two, or three); no projects
were rated high (eight to ten), and the remaining 20.3 percent
received ratings in the four to seven range.

MENTAL RETARDATION PROJECTS

The total group of 78 reports represents such a broad range of
disabilities and of rehabilitation efforts that further, more specific
statements are unfeasible. However, the 37 reports pertaining to
mental retardation seemed to be grouped into three fairly distinct
treatment approaches that were related to the level of disability served:
coordinated programs of special education and vocational rehabilitation
primarily within the school setting; sheltered workshops; and attempts
to upgrade the training of institutionalized retardates.

Coordinated Programs

The 19 projects concerned with cooperative special education/
vocational-rehabilitation programs served the adolescent and young
adult who generally could be considered an educable mentally retardate
(roughly, having an IQ of 50 to 75, although definitions varied and were

sometimes imprecise). The major components of these coordinated
programs were the following:

- Remedial attention (based on individual needs) to basic academic
  subjects, particularly reading, spelling, and arithmetic skills
- Occupation-related training: some combination of training within
  the educational setting and on-the-job training
- Attention to social and personal habits related to job success, in
  the form of care in placement, some type of counseling and support
  both preceding and during job placement, concern with work habits
  throughout all aspects of the program, and occasional attention to
  skills such as completing employment applications.

The major practical obstacles encountered by the programs
were staff problems (both lack of well-qualified staff and turnover)
and scarcity of appropriate placements (a problem frequently related
to community acceptance of the programs).

The 19 projects represent a trend in special education away from
a solely academic orientation and toward expanded vocational preparation. Another trend evident in some of these projects is the broadening of vocational training to include those of junior high school age
as well as young adults.

Within the limitations imposed by their typically poor research
methodology, some general conclusions about these 19 reports are
apparent. First, although such coordinated programs involve many
more problems than do programs with a strictly academic emphasis,
they are clearly feasible. Second, such programs appear to enhance
the employability of educable mentally retarded students. Their
degree of superiority over more academically oriented programs and
the optimum student population for them to serve remain to be demonstrated. Third, all three of the major components appear to be
essential; however, questions of relative emphasis remain to be
answered.

One of the better project reports was by Karnes et al. (1966).[*]
Since the students in the project were considered slow learners
(IQ 75 to 90) rather than educable mentally retarded, any generalization of results to the latter group should be made with caution. In
that coordinated special-education/vocational-rehabilitation program

---

[*]Karnes, M. B.; Zehrbach, R. R.; Jones, G. R.; MacGregor,
N. E.; George, J. M. "The Efficacy of a Prevocational Curriculum
and Services Designed to Rehabilitate Slow Learners Who are School
Dropout, Delinquency, and Unemployment Prone." (Champaign, Ill.:
Champaign Community Unit IV Schools, 1965).

the final sample consisted of 61 pairs of subjects (122 subjects)
matched on the basis of sex, race, SES, and IQ. Experimental subjects were provided with a vocationally-oriented educational program
and counseling, while controls were enrolled only in a regular educational program. The experimental group had significantly fewer
school dropouts, better attendance records, and better employment
records than the control group. There were no significant differences
in academic progress. Major methodological problems stemmed from
a rather large number of dropouts (especially from the control group),
a specially trained staff (which made it necessary to distinguish the
effect of the staff from that of the treatment variables), and no control
for Hawthorne effects.

Sheltered-Workshop Programs

Six of the projects in our sample serving the mentally retarded
employed the sheltered workshop approach. The populations they
served tended to be adult rather than of school age and were a more
severely retarded group, although the IQ ranges were in some instances
quite broad. The workshops endeavored to produce some type of quality
merchandise that could be marketed competitively, thereby providing
a means for training, employment, and some degree of client self-
sufficiency.

The concept of sheltered workshops is not new. A trend evident
in the six projects was their emphasis on evaluating clients by individual strengths and weaknesses. From a research standpoint, the
projects were neither well designed nor well evaluated. The reports,
mainly descriptive in nature, are valuable chiefly for their demonstrations of feasibility and for their dissemination of information
related to practical aspects of a sheltered workshop program.

Upgraded Institutional Training

Nine projects employed the third approach, which may loosely
be described as attempts to upgrade training for institutionalized
retarded populations. The subjects included in these projects were
apparently of a broad range of ages (ages often were not clearly specified); they tended to be severely or profoundly retarded (IQs below
approximately 35 are generally considered severe or profound retardation). In general, the services provided by the nine projects included
evaluation of potential for rehabilitation and heterogeneous types of

training designed to foster cognitive, social, and/or behavioral development. A variety of procedures was employed.

This group of reports illustrates the trend toward broadening the definition of special education to include training at whatever level is necessary to meet individual needs. The projects also represent the movement toward training programs and away from mere custodial care. Two general conclusions from this group of reports—their limitations notwithstanding—are that training can improve the status of the retarded population and that the success of training programs appears to depend upon both a careful assessment of needs and the development of individualized training programs.

The research methodology employed in the nine projects tended to be poor. Reliable measurement of variables with severely or profoundly retarded subjects is always difficult, and these projects were no exception. Staff problems were evident: staff members were often poorly trained and/or motivated. Although the superiority of a particular method—e.g., operant conditioning—over other training methods has been demonstrated elsewhere, that was generally not the concern of most of the projects. Future research would do well to address itself to the relative significance of specific kinds of training. The major value of the reports is in their description of evaluation procedures, types of training, and methods of training.

SUMMARY AND CONCLUSIONS

Although there were a few projects that were well planned and well executed, the overall quality of the projects we reviewed was disappointing. Sampling problems were frequent, control of variables tended to be poor, and research design and data analysis were generally unsophisticated. The chief value of the projects is their demonstration of the potential applicability of their methods. However, since their generalizability is limited, and since they made few conceptual or empirical contributions, we must give them a low rating in terms of policy utility.

It is hoped that in the future the emphasis will shift away from the present preponderantly descriptive research to more substantive investigations. The overall quality of projects needs much improvement if substantial contributions to rehabilitation practice are to be expected.

The discussion in this chapter focuses on a set of reports dealing with rehabilitation programs that are related to vocational education. Of the 59 project reports included, 91.5 percent dealt with the disciplines of vocational education or rehabilitation counseling. The remainder, although focusing primarily upon other disciplines, did entail some job-related services. The category of mental retardation represented the largest sample (22 out of 59, or approximately 37.3 percent) of any major disability focus of the projects. Other categories were orthopedic (13.6 percent), respiratory (6.8 percent), visually handicapped (5.1 percent), educationally and culturally disadvantaged (5.1 percent); the remainder of the projects were spread out over a number of other categories. In general, the reports discussed below fall in the framework of programs specifically designed or oriented toward a job-market approach or solution.

TREATMENT

As evidenced by the breakdown in Table 9.1, the treatment modalities employed in the set of projects point heavily toward vocationally-designed programs. The significant independent variables are vocational training and evaluation, placement services, on-the-job training, and sheltered workshops. Unfortunately, some

---

This chapter was written by Jerome J. Rosenberg, Associate Professor, Department of Special Education, Glassboro State College.

TABLE 9.1

Treatment or Independent Variables,
Vocational-Education Programs

Variable	Frequency
Vocational training	31
Evaluation	22
Placement services	21
Counseling	18
On-the-job training	14
Sheltered workshop setting	13
Medical treatment	5
Special education	4
Psychiatric help	3
Physical therapy	3
Team counseling	3
Evaluation (medical)	3
Speech therapy	2
Attitude changes	2
Outreach interviews	1
Halfway house	1
Social work (home visit)	1

difficulties exist with regard to various treatment techniques. A
review of the components of the treatment modalities indicated some
confusion about the definition of work evaluation. Work samples and
job samples are sometimes used interchangeably, causing further
confusion, especially with respect to job roles. Many facilities that
claimed to have provided "work adjustment" for their clients had
merely provided training without exposing the clients to real-life work
situations. In too many instances, after having received interviews,
a battery of psychological tests, and a 12- to 14-week work evaluation
program, clients went unaccounted for. Apparently, in many cases,
placement in a job was left to others, and it is impossible to learn of
the client's eventual success or lack of success in the job market.
Outcome measurements and follow-ups were often ignored.

In some projects the treatment was in the hands of a rehabilitation team that included a psychologist concerned with testing. Unfortunately, the battery of tests administered were sometimes interpreted
in a questionable manner. Too often, only final scores were obtained,
and no consideration was given to the client's reactions, the various

situations and conditions in which the tests were given, and so on. Most of the tests were constructed to predict success or the lack of failure in achieving the objectives of training, but test results must take into account the degree of variability in measurement and the client's situational characteristics.

The manual-dexterity aspects of the Purdue Pegboard, MRMT, WAIS, and so forth, appear to have a high correlation with job-sample tasks. But exclusive reliance on test results automatically eliminates some who might have succeeded. Job-task measurement is an imperfect predictor of success. Vocational evaluation should provide concrete descriptions of behavior, rather than diagnostic labels or phrases derived from imperfect testing programs.

A number of projects also relied heavily on the results of the vocational battery in their assessments of the clients' capabilities and interests. It is questionable whether those test results can be used to predict success in getting and keeping a job. The test results could be more useful if combined with the assignment of realistic work tasks in realistic work situations, something not often done in the project reports. There remains much room for improving the sophistication of diagnostic techniques in the field of rehabilitation. The disabled are a heterogeneous, not a homogeneous population, and hence, tests should attempt to distinguish significant differences between groups.

SAMPLE SIZE

The sample size (see Table 9.2) was generally in the 101 to 250 client range that appears to be an adequate basis for study in this type

TABLE 9.2

Sample Size, Vocational-Education Programs

Variable	Frequency
≤ 12	0
13-30	2
31-50	4
51-75	3
76-100	9
101-250	24
251-500	10
501 and over	6
Unknown	1

TABLE 9.3

Demographic, Rehabilitation-Related, and Socioeconomic Variables, Vocational-Education Programs

	Not Marked		Considered		Effects Analyzed		Partial or Weak Control		Strong Control	
	Number	Percent	Number	Percent	Number	Percent	Number	Percent	Number	Percent
Age	9	15.3	11	18.6	18	30.5	13	22.0	8	13.6
Sex	25	42.4	10	16.9	14	23.7	2	3.4	8	13.6
Residence	41	69.5	6	10.2	4	6.8	4	6.8	4	6.8
Race	51	86.4	3	5.1	5	8.5	0	0.0	0	0.0
Ethnicity	55	93.2	1	1.7	3	5.1	0	0.0	0	0.0
Religion	57	96.6	1	1.7	1	1.7	0	0.0	0	0.0
Intelligence	21	35.6	9	15.3	14	23.7	11	18.6	4	6.8
Education	30	50.8	8	13.6	14	23.7	2	3.4	5	8.5
Family structure	44	74.6	3	5.1	10	16.9	0	0.0	2	3.4
Type of disability	13	22.0	10	16.9	14	23.7	12	20.3	10	16.9
Duration of handicap	45	76.3	4	6.8	5	8.5	3	5.1	2	3.4
Severity of handicap	28	47.5	10	16.9	7	11.9	9	15.3	5	8.5
Previous institutional experience	46	78.0	6	10.2	4	6.8	1	1.7	2	3.4
Previous occupational experience	38	64.4	10	16.9	10	16.9	0	0.0	1	1.7
Previous military status	58	98.3	1	1.7	0	0.0	0	0.0	0	0.0
Income of client	53	89.8	1	1.7	4	6.8	1	1.7	0	0.0
Income of family	49	83.1	4	6.8	5	8.5	0	0.0	1	1.7
Social class	50	84.7	4	6.8	4	6.8	0	0.0	1	1.7
Occupation	48	81.4	5	8.5	5	8.5	0	0.0	1	1.7

of research; larger samples, however, would allow for greater variability of client type.

The frequency distributions of the demographic, rehabilitation-related, and socioeconomic variables discussed in this set of reports can be found in Table 9.3. Within each study, the variables provide a profile of the population under study. Of particular concern here is the apparent lack of interest in race, especially in the face of known labor-market discrimination on the basis of race. A similar lack of concern for socioeconomic variables would also appear to be a critical oversight.

METHODOLOGY

A design weakness that is common to much of this type of research and that detracts from the credibility of the statistical findings, stems from the identication and measurement of employment success. More than half of all the projects were concerned with the employability status of the clients at the outcome (see Table 9.4). Success criteria, as well as behavioral changes resulting from a variety of treatments, need to be studied. In many studies, the following measures were among those selected as reflecting employment success: whether clients found jobs on their own; whether the

TABLE 9.4

Outcome or Dependent Variables,
Vocational-Education Programs

Variable	Frequency
Employed/unemployed	33
Success/failure	10
Placed in a sheltered workshop	6
Rehabilitated/not rehabilitated	6
Test rating	4
Functioning capacity	4
On-the-job training	4
Client attitude change	2
Recidivism	2
Not applicable	1
Independent living style	1
Costs and benefits	1

individual held a job for at least two or three months; the total number
of hours worked; the total income earned; whether they had to be hospitalized or institutionalized. Yet those measures may be inadequate
as concepts of "success" in employment. There is still some doubt
whether those clients who were identified as successful were placed
in jobs in which they were efficient and well-adjusted and in which
they could look forward to long tenure.

Of particular interest were a number of studies dealing with
multiple-handicapped persons over the age of 35, a population that
traditionally has had a notable lack of success in vocational training
and placement. Although the projects appeared to be well-designed,
their objectives and goals were generally not attained. Older groups,
with previous records of disinterest and failure apparently need programs with intensive training and generous encouragement to rekindle
or, perhaps, to initially motivate them to succeed in a program of
occupational rehabilitation. For many of the clients success required
the gaining of acceptance and approval from someone with whom they
identified or someone who cared about them. The pattern was found
among projects that included the alcoholic, the parolee, the trainee
with a respiratory illness, the quadriplegic, and the mentally retarded.

STATISTICS AND DESIGN

Approximately half of the reports used some sort of statistical
procedure, but too many relied on simple presentation of data. The
reports also varied significantly with respect to experimental design.
Of the 59 projects reviewed, 23 (39 percent) were experimental in
design, and 36 (61 percent) were nonexperimental. Of the 23 experimental designs, 12 (52.2 percent) employed the one-shot case-study
design, four (17.4 percent) employed the one-group pretest/posttest
design, two (8.7 percent) employed the pretest/posttest control-group
design, and five (21.7 percent) reported other methods. The overall
ratings for the group of reports can be found in Table 9.5.

Although random sampling was often lacking, follow-ups
sketchy or nonexistent, statistical treatment of the data unsophisticated, and experimental design rather loose, there were still many
creative and important results that benefited a multitude of handicapped people. During our review of the literature, it became apparent
that several research projects, when confronted with problems, simply
gave up on research methodology and rationalized their continued use
of funds because of their provision of services to the handicapped.

Much of the research was generated and conducted in comparative
isolation, without reference to a larger theoretical framework. In only

TABLE 9.5

Policy-Utility and Methodology Rating,
Vocational-Education Programs

		Policy-Utility Rating		Methodology Rating	
		Tally	Percentages	Tally	Percentages
Low	1	1	1.7	0	0.0
	2	0	0.0	1	1.7
	3	2	3.4	4	6.8
	4	1	1.7	7	11.9
	5	2	3.4	11	18.6
	6	2	3.4	10	16.9
	7	6	10.2	3	5.1
	8	9	15.3	9	15.3
	9	11	18.6	4	6.8
High	10	25	42.4	10	16.9
Totals		59	100.0	59	100.0

a few instances was there an integrated and articulate series of
studies with a common theoretical focus. Those studies that concerned themselves with sound conceptual models of vocational behavior
and the testing of theoretical propositions were the ones that dealt with
the problems of measuring reinforcement, measuring satisfaction,
comparing groups, and validating test instruments.

Several projects focused on improving the self-concept and
work-adjustment attitudes of their clients. They isolated several
factors associated with job satisfaction—for example, personal adjustment, performance capability, emotional adjustment, family status,
economic status, travel to job, and so on. It was found that the clients
most likely to fail were those who had difficulty commuting to the job
(facility); troubled marital relations or poor family structure; multiple
handicaps; were over the age of 35; suffered economic hardship; or
lacked recognition for work well done. Those were the same factors
associated with job dissatisfaction and low self-esteem. Clients who
had had on-the-job training or work experience programs in an industrial setting evidenced improvements in both vocational and personal
outlook (Thompson et al., 1973; Goodman et al., 1967). It was also
found that clients improved significantly when they obtained satisfaction
in training positions; experienced psychological growth through chal-
lenging work activities; received their initial training in positions

where supervisors and coworkers were suitable role models and were individuals with whom they could interact; and entered their initial job with basic skills and specialized competencies that precluded failure and assured achievement, recognition, and responsibility.

The expectation in the projects was that the success experiences would be achieved in the sheltered setting and transferred to the outside world. The sheltered-workshop (on-campus) type of program in many instances does not have the impact of reality that is needed for the handicapped client's adjustment to the working world and to society. Clearly, a redirection in both training and types of programs is needed, if they are to prepare large numbers of trainees realistically for nonworkshop employment opportunities.

POLICY UTILITY

Because of our doubt about methodological adequacy, we cannot rely on results obtained with anything approximating absolute assurance. Some findings do emerge from a variety of projects. They should be considered when designing alternative programs for the handicapped. First, programs in rural areas face the difficulties of the unavailability of rehabilitation services, transportation, and job-placement agencies. Such difficulties are not faced by projects in high-density urban centers, but such centers are sometimes faced with more clients than can be served (Abbott, 1966; Mulhern, 1966). Second, workshops are sometimes used as a dumping ground; people are referred there just to give them a place to go. Third, the correction of the disability, in whole or in part after rehabilitation, appears minimal with multiple/severely handicapped. (For further discussion of the situation of the severely disabled the reader is referred to Chapter 12.) Fourth, industry-based work experiences have the impact of reality—an attribute of paramount importance in motivation and self-image of the client. Fifth, the mentally retarded tend to be placed in sheltered workshops more often than persons with other handicaps, who may be treated in community/industry facilities. Sixth, a planned program of industrial homework is useful for the severely disabled who are homebound (Kristeller and Stein, 1960; Jennings, 1963). Seventh, work potential can be increased, if secondary mental or physical dysfunctions are treated. Eighth, a greater degree of success is evidenced when vocational counselors maintain regular rather than sporadic contact with clients and employers. Ninth, once employers understand retardation, epilepsy, blindness, and so on, they become more highly motivated to employ the handicapped (Hewitt, 1967). Tenth, adjustment to competitive employment can be smooth and efficient after training in a simulated "real" industrial shop program. Finally, the primary flaws in the research methodology are lack of random sampling, inadequate methods to control for changes in the target population, poor selection of evaluators of the program, unsophisticated data collection devices and techniques, and lack of follow-up. The net result of those defects is the inability to generalize the findings to larger populations.

CONCLUSIONS

As this report has indicated, the special training needs of the handicapped remain unmet. Our society has not yet committed itself to the social and economic investment required in order to meet the training needs of larger numbers of handicapped people.

The literature regarding the mentally retarded is rife with statements from the leading specialists in the field to the effect that "the mentally retarded are more like us (non-handicapped) in learning, in feelings, than unlike us." Yet in practice the mentally retarded and the handicapped are not accorded the same treatment as normal persons; rather, they are perceived as both dependent and perpetually childlike.

Because the mentally retarded have been confined largely to the sheltered-workshop experience, a stereotype personality has emerged. It is an outgrowth of the consistent approval for conforming and behaving in a childlike and dependent manner. As a result, parents, legislators, employers, and counselors tend to view the workshop as a final placement for the handicapped.

Given the inadequacy of our present system of training, the reluctance of employers to hire the handicapped, and the overreliance of vocational-rehabilitation/special-education professionals upon the workshop setting, new directions are needed. Many suggestions have been made. These include the establishment of government as the employer of last resort. Alternatively, industry in cooperation with public programs could provide special funds for training, supervision, and services for the handicapped. That concept is endorsed by Ronald W. Conley, formerly of the Rehabilitation Services Administration of HEW, who maintains (Conley, 1974):

> Sheltered work opportunities should be developed in regular
> places of employment by reengineering jobs, paying less
> than standard wages, if necessary, shortening working
> hours, providing special supervision, etc. The immense
> diversity and productivity of American industry assures

that retardates so placed will normally earn far more
than they could earn in sheltered workshops.

Those kinds of programs are necessary if the handicapped are to avoid
the difficulties imposed by a culture that inhibits their change and
suppresses their individual differences. The very design of their
rehabilitation treatment is often retrogressive and dysfunctional.

SOME POSSIBILITIES FOR THE FUTURE

Placement of the mentally retarded in service jobs has had the
highest rate of success. Serious consideration should be given to
employing the handicapped in governmental facilities, especially if
civil service jobs and workloads were reassessed. There is a need
for new data and research in the vocational-rehabilitation field. For
example, we need to know more about why those who receive theoretically adequate services fail to attain their vocational potential. Perhaps, external factors, such as family life and community and work
environment, are significant here. In the overall effort to diminish
barriers to the employment of the handicapped, one possibility might
be an affirmative action plan for the handicapped, similar to that for
other minorities.

REFERENCES

Those reports noted by an asterisk were included in our sample
of 477 projects. A complete list of reports reviewed by the author is
available through the Disability and Health Economics Research Section.

*Abbott, W. M. "And Someday, Perhaps My Chance Will Come."
    Unpublished final report, Vocational Training Center, Inc.,
    Fargo, N.D., 1966.

Conley, R. W. Cited in Programs for the Handicapped. Washington,
    D.C.: Office of Mental Retardation, January 30, 1974.

*Goodman, S. M., Caldwell, A. W., Floyd, R. F., et al. The Work
    Oriented Curriculum Project. Rockville, Md.: Montgomery
    County Public Schools, Educational Services Center, 1967.

*Hewitt, D. W. "Work Inc.: A Demonstration of Personal Adjustment
    and Intensive Placement Techniques with Difficult to Place Dis-
    abled People in an Area of High Unemployment Incidence."
    Unpublished final report, Division of Vocational Rehabilitation,
    Tallahassee, Fla., 1967.

*Jennings, R. "Working Competitively at Home." Unpublished final
    report, Detroit League for the Handicapped, Inc., Detroit,
    Mich., 1963.

*Kristeller, E. L., and Stein, L. L. "The Rehabilitation of Poten-
    tially Employable Homebound Adults." Unpublished final report,
    New York University, Bellevue Medical Center, N.Y., 1960.

*Mulhern, F. P. "Work Adjustment and Evaluation Center for Older
    Disabled Workers." Unpublished final report, Mankato Rehabil-
    itation Center, Inc., Mankato, Minn., 1966.

*Thompson, N. M., Farbish, G., and Hefley, R. J. An Evaluation
    of a Prevocational Adjustment Program for Low Income Women.
    Houston, Tex.: Neighborhood Centers Day Care Association,
    1973.

10

PSYCHIATRIC
REHABILITATION

This chapter focuses on studies dealing with the rehabilitation of the mentally ill, with special emphasis on the plight of individuals after their release from psychiatric hospitals. The 20 studies reviewed dealt mainly with two problematic aspects of the ex-patients' situation: vocational training and transitional living arrangements. Several of the studies covered both of these areas. A number of reports concerned settings in which transitional living situations included vocational training as a major part of the program. The major orientation of all the reports is treatment aimed at community adjustment; self-sufficient return to community living is specifically noted in many of the reports as a general measure of success. Reflecting this goal, most of the programs are marked by interaction with the community through volunteer participation or community placement of clients.

While the reports are obviously of interest to administrators and researchers in the mental health field, they may be also of use to anyone who deals with individuals who have been removed from society and require assistance to return successfully. Many of the techniques utilized would appear to have good generalizability for other areas of disability.

––––––––––––

This chapter was written by Julius Lanoil, Director of Psychiatric Rehabilitation, Rutgers Community Mental Health Center, and Daniel M. Roddick, Research Associate, Psychiatric Rehabilitation, RCMHC. A complete list of the reports reviewed by these authors is available from the Disability and Health Economics Research Section.

INTERNAL VALIDITY

In general, the methodology of the studies considered in this chapter was not of a high level: 30 percent were rated in the lowest possible category evaluating overall methodology; only 5 percent were rated in the highest category (see Table 10.1).

TABLE 10.1

Gross Methodology Ratings,
Psychiatric-Rehabilitation Reports

	Poor . . . . Very Good									
	1	2	3	4	5	6	7	8	9	10
90	30	5	15	5	15	10	0	10	5	5
N	6	1	3	1	3	2	0	2	1	1

Closer examination reveals the following specific areas of methodological weakness:

Sampling

Largely because of a combination of inadequate representativeness and drawing procedure, 68.2 percent were found to be of doubtful generalizability. Sample sizes were marginally acceptable, with the modal size falling at about 80 individuals. Dropouts were handled poorly in about one-third of the studies. That weakness in research methodology is, of course, unequalled in its potential for distortion of outcome measures. Frequent serious problems of highly restrictive screening resulted in samples that were unrepresentative in terms of the general population of persons leaving mental hospitals.

Research Design

Herein lies the real problem with the attempt to evaluate the methodology of the studies. In many cases, the treatment activities

described in the studies were not established for research purposes
but rather for the sole purpose of handling the needs of the expatient.
That exclusive service orientation creates two problems. First, few
of the projects included a control group (35.7 percent), and many were
without a clear hypothesis (37.4 percent). Alternative hypotheses were
presented in only 19.4 percent of the studies. These and other design
weaknesses make evaluation or comparison of programs very difficult.
As stated before, however, those shortcomings are to be expected in
projects that were designed merely to meet a specific need in an
existing program. The second problem is that many of the design
problems are accentuated when researchers attempt to accommodate
to them. There are frequent attempts to bend a successfully operating
program into an experimental design, resulting in a project description that may detract from the basic quality of the project concept.
Over half of the studies were found by the checklisters to be unusable
or questionable for general use because of either poor methodology
or unclear reporting or both.

Statistics

The statistical procedures in the group of studies were generally
low-powered. Most used simple correlational analysis (82 percent),
with only 9 percent utilizing techniques such as multivariate analysis.
The complexity of the factors involved in these projects would indicate
that more careful design would have included the production of data
that could be analyzed in a more sophisticated manner.

Other Areas of Methodological Concern

No mention of follow-up was made in 71.4 percent (N = 15) of
the reports. The lack is compounded by the rather short time periods
clients were observed (mode equaled three to six months). The follow-
up is an absolutely essential element in the type of study reviewed.
Success figures cannot be based upon "number of clients returning to
full-time employment," since the fact of return is not the issue;
rather, it is the duration of return. Extensive and lengthy follow-up
studies are the only source of that key information.

THE FOUNTAIN HOUSE PROJECT

We have selected one of the studies included in this chapter for closer review in order to illustrate its good methodology and its raising of an important question that could have high policy utility. Although it exemplifies some of the better works examined, it also evidences one of the typical problems of research in the area—i.e., lack of long-term follow-up (in this case attributable to the funding service).

The project, "An Evaluation of Rehabilitation Services and the Role of Industry in the Community Adjustment of Psychiatric Patients Following Hospitalization," took place at the Fountain House Foundation in New York City. It was directed by James R. Schmidt and reported in July 1969. The purpose of the study was to "determine the extent to which private enterprise could participate in the vocational rehabilitation of discharged psychiatric patients and evaluate the effects of rehabilitation services on the community adjustment of such subjects." A group of 202 subjects were screened by several criteria, including age, number of hospitalizations, and employment status (must be unemployed) and were randomly assigned to three groups:

Control group: After an interview in which they were informed that Fountain House could not accept all applicants, the subjects were told that there were no openings available for them.

Community placement service group. After a similar interview, the subjects were referred to a local community service offering the services of a vocational counselor.

Fountain House group. After being interviewed, these subjects were accepted for the Fountain House Program, which included several types of services: personal adjustment training, social and recreational programs, a transitional employment program, an apartment program, and a job placement service.

The focus of the study was primarily on the transitional-employment program and the feasibility of intimate involvement of the community in the rehabilitation process. Jobs in business and industry were taken on by the program and were then filled by program participants, who were carefully matched with the job and trained under the supervision of the Fountain House staff. Jobs were divided into half-time or smaller time blocks, depending upon the situation of each worker. Individuals could stay on jobs for a number of months before moving to another position, or they could leave a job after a very short time, if the move was necessary. The employer was

guaranteed continuity, however, because the program provided un-
broken coverage of the job.

During that particular study, 40 firms participated and made
work opportunities available in 160 positions, at an annual combined
wage of more than $300,000 for the year.

All subjects in the study were evaluated over a period of 18
months on their rates of employment, agency contacts, rehospitaliza-
tions and other factors. The results, as in many of the studies, were
somewhat difficult to interpret. For instance, a factor like rehospitalization rates is very ambiguous: Subjects not in a program have
understandably fewer contacts with mental-health workers, and that
fact may clearly affect rehospitalization rates or the length of time
between the development of certain symptoms or situations and the
return to the hospital.

Briefly, the results were as follows: First, the rate of rehospitalization for the Fountain House group was lower than that for the
other two groups but not to a statistically significant extent. Statistical significance for that factor was found, however, for subjects
who entered the program within four months of their release from
the hospital. Second, the total person-days employed for the Fountain
House group were 10,430; for the community placement services
group they were 7,940, and for the control group, 8,543. Third, 86
percent of the Fountain House group were placed in a position, compared to a 57-percent figure for each of the other two groups.

Many of the studies we reviewed reported much more spectacu-
lar success rates than those, but the results could often be traced to
some technique that may have distorted the outcome. The strength of
the study lies in its careful design and conservative evaluation of
results.

The major weakness of the Fountain House project, as noted by
the researchers, was its short time span: Posthospital adjustment
cannot be considered adequately in only 18 months. Long-term panel
studies clearly hold the most promise for accurate and consistent
results.

The Fountain House project on transitional employment stands,
then, as a carefully constructed experimental situation that, although
not recording any remarkable success statistics, does afford a detailed account of a technique that has both a good theoretical basis
and high policy utility.

POLICY UTILITY

So much is needed by individuals who are entering the community from mental hospitals and who are deprived of social,

vocational, residential, and educational alternatives, that it becomes
difficult to criticize any effort that attempts to ease their adjustment.
Nevertheless, certain future directions seem clear.

First, in the area of vocational rehabilitation, ways must be
found to involve the business community so that people returning from
the hospital can participate in real-work situations in the community.
That kind of work situation is necessary, regardless of the type of
prevocational program, if the person is to move on to normalcy. One
of the best studies in the area in terms of methodology, done at the
Fort Logan Mental Health Center demonstrated that the offering of a
sheltered workshop without any community placement produced no
statistically significant effect on later vocational adjustment, regardless of how well the individual did within the workshop itself.*
Judging by the studies we reviewed, those programs offering graduated
work experiences within the facility and in the community, offer the
highest policy utility potential. Programs must attempt to maintain
support for many persons, even after full-time employment is achieved
Obviously, since long-term support is necessary for so many of the
people, short-term, high-expectancy programs will not do the job.

Second, many studies shared a common weakness of focusing
on a single dimension of a person's life. One must consider the total
human being and must be aware that he or she will grow to the extent
that social, vocational, residential, and educational opportunities
are offered. Focusing on one to the exclusion of all others is like
supplying a person with only part of his daily vitamin requirement for
survival. That was true for many of the halfway-house demonstration
projects, which offered social and residential programs but did little
in terms of vocational training.

Third, although there was only one study in our sample concerning multiple-disability, † it is interesting to note that individuals
referred for psychiatric rehabilitation through a hearing-rehabilitation
center were accepted and received the psychiatric services at a level
equal with other clients.

Fourth, psychiatric rehabilitation has traditionally been kept
separate from the medical treatment of schizophrenia, but it becomes
extremely important, in an administrating rehabilitation program, to

---

*McDonald and Miles, "Evaluation of Work as Therapy for
Psychiatric Patients," (Denver, Colorado: Fort Logan Mental Health
Center, 1969).

†J.D. Rainer, and K.Z. Altshuler, <u>Comprehensive Mental Health
Services for the Deaf</u>, final report (New York: New York State Psychiatric Institute, 1966).

see to it that clients receive appropriate medication. Recognition of
medical treatment is particularly important with reference to any
evaluative research on rehabilitation. The factor of medication is
such a powerful variable that program developers must be extremely
sensitive to its implications for the program's success. Close communication should therefore be established between the medical and
rehabilitation people so as to closely coordinate the individual's upward
movement in the rehabilitation program and keep it consistent with
the changes in medication. The medication versus social-therapy
debate no longer seems relevant, given our present understanding of
the schizophrenic's fear of success. A two-pronged treatment—therapy
and medication—is critical.

RECOMMENDATIONS

All studies and programs should have a long-term follow-up
potential built in. This corresponds to our recommendations that
programs dealing with the posthospitalized patients should have no
time limit. The supports may be necessary for a long period of time
in whatever phase of a program a person is in.

Rehabilitation programs must provide feasible and relevant
social, vocational, residential, and educational components and must
have strong liaison with medical personnel to assure the administration of proper medication.

Future researchers should attempt to develop new and innovative
ideas, rather than over-research old ones.

The delivery of services in the area of psychiatric rehabilitation
cannot be equated with the delivery of services for physical disability.
The success of psychiatric rehabilitation is not as readily identifiable
as in many cases of physical rehabilitation. Programs that fail to
recognize that crucial difference will tend to focus on factors that are
not really essential to the recovery process.

Finally, if we recognize the dynamics of fear of success and
the extraordinary motivational problems that many of these people
have, we must realize that all program techniques are merely tools
to be used by the staff in their effort to establish relationships that
will help them improve patient motivation. It is on this staff-patient
relationship that we must focus.

**CORRELATES OF
SUCCESS AND
PREDICTION OF
OUTCOMES**

This chapter reviews a number of studies that analyze the factors associated with success or failure in rehabilitation. The studies cross several disciplines, and unlike other groups of studies they do not focus on one method of rehabilitation treatment or on a single handicap. The typical study examines the outcomes of some relevant program over a period of time and seeks to determine whether it is possible to discriminate between successful and unsuccessful rehabilitation clients on the basis of socioeconomic, demographic, or treatment variables.

The notion of being able to identify the correlates of success in rehabilitation has an obvious appeal. If one can validly associate certain applicant characteristics with success, one can apply the knowledge to the selection process. It would also be possible to weigh case closures, based on indexes of difficulty generated by the research.

We examined 75 studies that attempted to predict rehabilitation outcome or to measure correlates of success. In addition, we examined 15 pieces of research that are directly related to outcomes studies—for example, scales of rehabilitation gain and measurement of outcome variables, reviews of the literature, and so on. Table 11.1 presents a breakdown of the major disabilities examined in the 75

The authors would like to thank Stanford E. Rubin of the University of Arkansas R&T Center, M. S. Tseng of the West Virginia University R&T Center, and Lowell Lenhart of the Department of Institutions, SRS, Oklahoma, for the publications they made available to the Bureau of Economic Research. Leo A. Micek of the Colorado Department of Social Services kindly answered questions about his research.

TABLE 11.1

Disability Groups Addressed in Correlates
of Success and Prediction of Outcomes

Disability	Number of Studies
Mental illness	20
Mental retardation	8
Mixed physical and mental	29
Physical	17
Social	1
Total	75

Note: Only 20 of the 75 research reports were part of our
sample of 477 reports. As indicated in Chapter 1, we added reports
in the area of correlates of success because of our special interest
in the area.

studies under consideration. The research efforts have varied with
respect to the quality of the research, the methodology employed,
and the usefulness of the results. They also vary with respect to
specific disability examined within major disability groups. For
example, the physical disability category in Table 11.1 lists 17 research projects; those may be subdivided into seven studies of mixed
physical disabilities: two studies each of hemiplegics, deafness, and
spinal cord dysfunction, and one study each of blindness, epilepsy,
heart-attack victims, and tuberculosis.

Before focusing on the specifics of methodology and policy
utility, we shall examine several general conclusions which emerge
from the body of research. First, while in some rehabilitation settings
investigators have been quite successful in their attempts to differen-
tiate between rehabilitants and nonrehabilitants, the majority of researchers have reported only modest predictive power. Second, while
many variables have been linked to rehabilitation success, there are
conflicting reports in the literature on the relationship between certain
variables and rehabilitation success (Westerheide and Lenhart, 1974,
pp. 10-16). We suspect that many of the apparent inconsistencies
result from the application of different methodologies to different
disabilities under investigation, and from the differential use of outcome measures, independent variables, and time dimensions.* Third,

---

*Among the many outcomes considered are acceptance or
rejection for services, completion or noncompletion of rehabilitation

among the characteristics often cited as being correlated with success are age (younger) race (white), education (higher), and marital status (married). Those variables are also significant in studies of labor-force participation; and, since employment is a common measure of rehabilitation program success, we might expect to find them significant in rehabilitation outcome studies. Fourth, a review of the literature indicates that there does not appear to be a uniform theoretical model of rehabilitation outcome; there are, however attempts to specif causality, as evidenced by models that include treatment variables. The fact that there is no universally accepted theoretical model of rehabilitation is not surprising; it does not necessarily follow that clients with different disabilities could be rehabilitated with similar treatments. Research within a given disability is generally based upon different models. In other words, researchers investigating the outcomes of the mentally retarded might not use the same variables or statistical methods. That could be a reflection of the different rehabilitation settings they are using to generate data, the way they perceive the rehabilitation process, or a combination of those and other factors. Finally there has not been a systematic attempt to measure the correlates of success and to predict rehabilitation outcome using a national random sample of the population of potential rehabilitants.

While those broad conclusions do not paint the most promising picture, there is much that can be done to improve research in the area, and the consequent potential for policy utility is vast.

QUALITY OF RESEARCH UNDERTAKEN

There were many strong points to the research we evaluated, possibly due to the fact that 53 of the 75 studies came to us from journals.* It would seem that journal publication serves as a screening mechanism, weeding out the grossest errors.

------

program, employment or unemployment at follow-up, and release from or retention in an institutional setting.

*The breakdown is mental illness, 16; mental retardation, 5; mixed physical and mental, 19; and physical 13. Social disability will be subsumed in the mixed category for this and subsequent analysis.

Sampling

Despite the preponderance of journal research, we found that sampling was not of a high caliber. Nearly every report describes the "sample" or subjects under investigation, including the numbers involved. Most describe the selection process, but a few do not. There were only eight random samples cited in the 75 reports.* That was not unexpected, however, since most of the projects were involved with populations that were readily adaptable to statistical manipulation, and, therefore, the need for random sampling was eliminated. One would assume that the investigators of smaller populations would be loath to lose observations, yet the most common fault in the "sampling" was the screening out of cases. On some occasions that was done for practical reasons—e.g. all those over age 60 were screened out, because their labor market opportunities, and hence by some measurements their vocational rehabilitation potential, were limited. One study screened out all those without a telephone; if part of a population without a telephone is comprised of a group with common characteristics (low income, young, single, and so on), the biasing effects are obvious. Regardless of the reasons for screening out cases, omissions will limit generalizability.

Dropouts, Refusals, and Nonresponses

Dropouts, refusals and nonresponses in the study sample may also influence results. If, as a group, they do not vary systematically from a study's active participants, their statistical treatment is not important; however, the fact that they are nonparticipants presents a prima facie case that they do differ from the study group. Much of the research on the prediction of rehabilitation outcomes presents the null hypothesis that there is no difference between successful and unsuccessful rehabilitation clients. The investigator then attempts to discriminate between the two groups. In general, although dropouts are treated as failures and are explicitly accounted for in the research, there is seldom any mention of refusals or nonresponses. Much of the research is retrospective and is likely to have been conducted by a third party who has gathered the working data from a completed

---

*Mental retardation, 1; mixed mental and physical, 5; and physical, 2.

project. The investigator may, then, be uncertain as to the number of those who were referred to but refused participation in the rehabilitation project. We can only speculate about the effects upon research quality of the failure to account for refusals and nonresponses.

PREDICTION AND ESTIMATION BASED ON
SCREENED SAMPLES

Much prediction and estimation is done on samples that have been selected by counselors. That is a problem with conceptual similarities to those discussed above, and it seems to be marked by the absence of its consideration in the literature. The policy implications of failing to consider problems introduced by the use of samples that have been chosen by counselors could be great. We shall treat it here, however, since its origins are methodological.

Multivariate statistical techniques have frequently been recommended as a tool to aid counselors in deciding whom to accept or reject for rehabilitation services. A somewhat less frequent suggestion has been to base that decision completely upon statistical determination. (Sawyer, 1966, p. 192; Campbell and Stanley, 1963, p. 63.) Researchers who recommend a multiple correlation technique may be correct in assuming that it will enable them to predict outcomes with greater accuracy than counselors; however, the existing research in the rehabilitation-outcome literature does not generally bear out that assumption. For example, let us consider a piece of research in which data are gathered from a state vocational-rehabilitation agency and the clients are dichotomized based upon the criterion of successful or unsuccessful rehabilitation. A multiple linear regression might be run on the dichotomy with the expectation that the resulting coefficients estimated will then be applied to the characteristics of future applicants for the program in order to arrive at an estimate of their conditional probability of successful rehabilitation. (The statistical difficulties with this technique will be discussed later.) Invariably, the coefficients estimated are derived from a "sample" of those clients already accepted into a vocational-rehabilitation program, but the rehabilitation counselors may have screened out close to half of the referrals as not acceptable for services. In applying the coefficients estimated from the "sample" to a potential applicant we would, in effect, be saying that the probability of his successful completion of the program, <u>given</u> acceptance, is identical to the probability of successful completion for the population at risk. Only if we were to assume that counselors randomly screen clients, would this procedure be justifiable. (We might note as an aside that attempts at cross validation are subject to the same difficulty, since the validating sample will probably be conditioned by acceptance.)

In citing the multiple regression technique for illustrative purposes we do not mean to imply that the problem is a function of the statistical tool used. In fact, Grigg, Holtman, and Martin (1970) made good use of the technique in estimating, first, the probability of acceptance into the rehabilitation program and, then, with the same variables, the probability of completing it successfully. Certainly, that a partial circumvention of the difficulty mentioned above.

Obviously, outcome studies will have to be expanded in order to account for the counselor screening before they can be touted as the ultimate selection device. But at present they are unquestionably valuable in alerting rehabilitation practitioners to differential client needs. Outcome studies are also applicable to situations (e.g., institutional settings) where questions of acceptance or rejection are moot. In such a setting one may attempt to estimate the probability of successful rehabilitation of, say, coronary recovery, without having to consider the biasing effect of screening.

Cross Validation

Although random sampling is not a requisite, given the population sizes, it would have been advisable to have had random assignment of subjects to a study group and a cross-validation or replication group. Only six of the 75 studies employed cross validation or replication, although some others discussed the need for cross validation. One study (De Mann, 1963, p. 340) employed cross validation in time, using as a normative group those cases "accepted for services between July 1, 1953, and June 30, 1956, and closed by July 1, 1959. An extension in time validation group . . . whose cases were accepted for services between July 1, 1956, and June 30, 1958, and closed by July 1, 1959."

Efforts to cross validate over time should be strongly encouraged. And cross validations at a point in time are also needed. It would be preferable to validate on completely independent samples; however, even validation on half-samples randomly assigned would be a welcome addition to the field of rehabilitation research.

Experimental Design

Some rehabilitation research projects are experimental in nature, and others lend themselves quite easily to true experimental designs. However, that is not the case when attempts are made to predict rehabilitation outcomes.

Some of the outcome studies we reviewed were similar to Campbell and Stanley's quasi-experimental Regression-Discontinuity Analysis (Campbell and Stanley, 1966, p. 61). But many were neither experimental nor quasi-experimental in nature. As can be surmised from our discussion on cross validation, control groups were seldom used in the research, and controls, when they were established, were usually the result of multivariate technique rather than by experimental design.

Statistical Techniques

As opposed to so much of the research reported on in this study (see Chapters 4 and 6), the statistical tools applied in the prediction of rehabilitation outcomes and correlates of success were often quite sophisticated. It is a truism that the nature of the data "dictates the type of statistical technique applied" (McNemar, 1969, p. 431). It is also evident that the very nature of the research we are examining requires that the investigator apply statistical tools. Table 11.2 provides some idea of the breadth of techniques applied in the research.

That the assumptions underlying the use of the various statistical tools were seldom discussed is probably a reflection of the researchers' perception of their audience. (However, there were exceptions; see Gilbert and Lester [1970].) More than half of the studies we examined were journal publications, and it is therefore to be expected that the researchers, in addressing their colleagues, would not see fit to include a review of basic statistics.

In general, the tests were correctly applied. For example, the point biserial correlation was reported in cases where the researcher was dealing with what he regarded as a true dichotomy, and the biserial correlation was reported when he believed the dichotomy represented a truly continuous variable. There were some questionable decisions made, however. For example, in establishing controls, it would appear to be imperative to employ multivariate techniques in prediction studies, but such techniques were often bypassed. A single variable (e.g., that the age of unsuccessful clients was greater than that of successful clients) does not meet policy-utility needs, nor does it meet with methodological standards. We need to know something about the other characteristics of the clients and about the interaction of their attributes. Similarly, when the setting justifies it, one-way analysis of variance (ANOVA) should not be accepted

TABLE 11.2

Some Techniques and Tests Applied in Correlates of
Success and Prediction of Outcomes

Technique or Test	Number of Studies
Multiple regression	19[a]
Factor analysis	9[b]
Discriminant-function analysis	7
Analysis of variance	18[c]
Product-moment correlation	12
Point-biserial correlation	4[d]
Biserial correlation	3
Phi coefficient	2
Partial correlation	2
Correlation (type unspecified)	4
t tests	17
Chi-square tests	21
Other nonparametric tests	9
No tests	3

[a]Includes stepwise regression.
[b]Includes two cases of principle components.
[c]Includes two nonparametric ANOVA.
[d]Includes one multiple-point biserial.

in place of two-way analysis with interactions and simple correlation
should not be substituted for multiple correlation. (The Arkansas
R&T Center has been interested in counselor-client interaction and
has developed a two-way model; see Rubin, Bolton, and Salley [1973].)
 Whereas several researchers did not make the most out of
their available data, others attempted to do so but, in so doing,
made errors. A common error arose in cases where multiple regression was run with a dichotomous dependent variable.* Eight

---

*When the dependent variable is a dichotomy, the application
of ordinary least squares will yield results that may be interpreted
as the conditional probability of an event, given the set of independent
variables. The regression coefficients estimated are unbiased
(assuming the model is correctly specified or at least that the re-
gressors are orthogonal—not a likely event); however, the error
term varies systematically with the dependent variable and,

studies reported t statistics for regression coefficients or reported R^2. Unfortunately, since the researchers were unaware that their statistics were invalid, they were reported without caveats. In one instance an investigator who was aware of the pitfalls of the technique pointed out the existence of heteroskedasticity and avoided the use of the classic statistical tests. He mentioned as a possible circumvention of the problem the application of generalized least squares (Bellante, 1972, p. 229).

We did not find a single attempt to avoid the problem through the use of probit analysis, logit analysis, or a maximum-likelihood technique. In fairness, it should be pointed out that those investigators who choose discriminant-function analysis (and possibly other techniques) may have done so because they wished to avoid the problems introduced by multiple regression on dichotomies. (Toms and Brewer [1971] and Peck and Stephens [1964] were aware that they were avoiding the problem by choosing another technique.)

The foregoing does not mean to imply that multiple regression should not be used in research when the dependent variable may only be 0 or 1. In fact, the conditional probabilities derived from the application of the technique may allow for accurate classification and prediction. Some of the research that contains the flaw is still valuable, both for predictive purposes and for the estimation of individual coefficients. There are other practical reasons that would lead researchers to use multiple-regression techniques over methodologically sounder techniques:*

1. The use of multiple regression is far less costly than a technique like a probit. Models estimated with probit at Rutgers University have cost approximately four times as much as regression; generalized least squares have cost twice as much.

---

consequently, with the independent variables. Heteroskedasticity is present (Goldberger, p. 249). The estimates derived will be inefficient, and the estimated standard errors will not be consistent. The standard tests of significance do not apply (Nerlove and Press, 1973, pp. 5-7). In addition, R^2 does not have the usual interpretation (Morrison, 1972, pp. 68-70; Neter and Maynes, 1970, pp. 501-09). Finally, although probabilities are bounded by zero and one, predictions generated by the technique under consideration can be negative or greater than one.

*We are indebted to Frederick C. Collignon of the University of California at Berkeley for calling these points to our attention.

2. Regression results, while not uncomplicated, are easier to explain
   to a lay audience, and authors are justifiably concerned with reporting their results in understandable form.
3. The sophisticated computer programs necessary to employ advanced techniques are not yet readily available to the rehabilitation-research community.
4. Although estimated probabilities may fall outside the 0-to-1 bounds,
   researchers can simply interpret those estimates that are greater
   than 1 as highly likely events and those less than 0 as highly im-
   probable events. Similarly, although estimated standard errors
   are biased, they are biased upwards. In other words, t statistics,
   which are not technically correct as reported, may be seen as
   conservative.

Measurement of Rehabilitation Gain

The rehabilitation literature contains frequent criticisms of the
inadequacy of closure 26 as a measure of success and of closure 28
or 30 as a reflection of failure (see Lenhart et al., 1972). The
criticism certainly has merit: Obviously, the success/failure dichotomy does not capture the many gains derived from a rehabilitation
program. If someone is exposed to a vocational rehabilitation model
but is closed as nonrehabilitated, it does not follow that neither he
nor society benefitted from his exposure. In fact, there is no way to
quantify the gains occurring in such cases. Several research efforts
have attempted to develop measures of benefit that reflect gain either
as a continuous or some other nondichotomous variable (Westerheide
and Lenhart, 1973; Lenhart et al. 1972; Reagles, Wright, and Butler,
1970a, 1970b). Such research has great potential policy utility, and
its expansion could change the nature of prediction studies. Be that
as it may, we shall continue to be interested in dichotomies, such
as employed/unemployed, so long as Congress continues to cite
employability as a criterion for admission into the federal-state rehabilitation program.

Interpretation of Factors

Besides the measurement problems encountered in the literature,
there are problems of interpretation. Factor analysis, a technique
that has been used in some studies, is especially useful in situations
where the researcher is confronted with many variables. However,

there is a danger that, in its application, the researcher will
"interpret" the factors as if they were a single variable or a single
attribute. It is true that some factors may contain attributes that
are so similar that they can be interpreted as a single variable. But
some researchers have stretched their imagination (and their readers'
credulity) with elaborate and poorly reasoned definitions of their
factors. If a factor comprises many heterogeneous variables, its
usefulness is limited both for prediction and for manipulation by
practitioners. Even if the factors are homogeneous in content, their
use will be limited, if they are loaded by exotic test scores or by
variables that will be difficult to obtain for rehabilitation applicants.

Despite the shortcomings of some the research efforts, we
would close this section with the observation that we did have some
substantive research to review. "Samples" were reported, hypotheses
tested, and statistical tools applied. The fact that much of the research was presented for journal publication and peer review assures
at least a modicum of research respectability. We shall shortly
discuss several of the studies we reviewed.

POLICY UTILITY

With so many of these research efforts being funded by tax
dollars, we might well ask ourselves why we are devoting tax money
to the prediction of rehabilitation outcomes or to the measurement
of the correlates of success. The answer can be divided into the
following major categories, each of which we shall consider in turn:
planning and the allocation of resources; insurance and actuarial
purposes; and an adjunct to the development of a weighted case closure
scheme.

Planning and Resource Allocation

At the national level, if we had accurate estimates of the
probability of successful rehabilitation stratified by age, race, sex,
disability, and relevant treatment and control variables, we could
apply those data to the projected social benefits and costs accruing
to the rehabilitation of identical stratified subsets. The result would
be a picture of the differential social rates of return on our investment in human capital. (The methodology described here has been
employed in Bellante [1972].) We could use those rates of return as
guides for differential funding patterns in an attempt to maximize the

return on our social investment. If we assume that the probability
estimates are valid over time—and this may be a reasonable assumption for short periods (Sinnett et al. [1965] makes the point that
different variables may influence rehabilitation in the long run and
in the short run)—we may use them together with population projec-
tions and disability incidence rates to forecast social-service needs,
program budgets, training requirements, and dependency states for
various populations at risk.

Analogously, at a local or district level there are limited
resources to be allocated. When one considers that there are probably
more individuals in need of rehabilitation services than can be served,
given budget constraints, it is evident that attention must be directed
to selecting the case mix that maximizes allocative efficiency (see
Miller and Allen, 1966, p. 349; Burstein et al., 1965, p. 127; Novis
et al., 1960, p. 267). In some rehabilitation settings (e.g., in mental
hospitals and in programs where the number of potential trainees
exceeded the number of training slots available) it would be especially
beneficial to rank clients by their degree of readiness for training
(see Brooks and Weaver, 1965, p. 71).

Insurance and Actuarial Purposes

If we combine the probability of successful rehabilitation with
data on the probability of becoming disabled, we can obtain valuable
information on the public's insurance needs. That expanded information can contribute to market efficiency, improving either a public
or private market for rehabilitation insurance.

It may be possible to view rehabilitation service as an entitlement. (We might wish to provide rehabilitation services to all those
who apply, or we might guarantee services to those applicants whose
probability of success indicates economic efficiency.) Under our
current system, in which the rehabilitation counselor determines a
client's acceptability, the correlates of success could aid appreciably
in making that determination, thereby saving valuable counselor time
(Novis et al., 1960). As noted above, we could also use those measures in selecting those clients who are in need of the most intensive
services (Bolton, 1972; Tseng, 1972; De Mann, 1963).

Development of a Weighted Case Closure

The time, effort, and resources devoted to rehabilitating a
client vary with the socioeconomic, demographic, and disability

characteristics he brings to the rehabilitation setting. In order to evaluate programs we must be able to distinguish among cases on the basis of difficulty (Lenhart et al., 1972, p. 29). For example, we might compare "expected outcome" (probability of success) with "actual outcome" to evaluate program performance (Stein et al., 1970, p. 95; Noble [1973] makes an analogous point). If we find that an agency has accepted a particularly difficult case mix, we will have something more substantial than the number of 26-case closures with which to gauge their efficiency.

The above considerations represent only a partial list of the actual and potential policy-utility benefits flowing from research on rehabilitation outcomes. Since those benefits have direct impact upon rehabilitation practice, the allocation of rehabilitation resources, and the lives of rehabilitation clients, it is imperative that such research be both methodologically sound and widely disseminated. We shall now examine several research efforts that we consider to be important methodologically, conceptually, for reasons of policy utility, or for a combination of those.

REVIEW OF KEY PROJECTS

There are several sources that the interested reader should consult for a review of the literature (Westerheide and Lenhart, 1974; Rubin, Bolton, and Salley 1973; Rubin and Salley, 1973; Cobb, 1972; Segal, 1972; Day et al., 1969; Hammond, Wright, and Butler, 1968).

We shall devote our attention here to four research efforts that, in our opinion, are better methodologically than most prediction research, although they are not without flaws. They are not isolated pieces of quality research; we could well have chosen others and, in fact, found it difficult to limit ourselves to four.

The first piece examined, a journal article, was not sponsored research—i.e., it listed no sponsor. The second piece was sponsored by the Vocational Rehabilitation Administration, HEW; the third piece, by the Cooperative Research Program of the Office of Education, HEW; the fourth, by SRS.

Toms and Brewer, 1971

A population of 239 former mental patients who had applied for vocational rehabilitation while hospitalized was trichotomized. Group I (N_1 = 54) was composed of discharged patients who had received no vocational services. Group II (N_2 = 90) consisted of discharged patients who received VR services but were closed as not rehabilitated. Group III (N_3 = 95) contained those discharged patients who received services and were closed rehabilitated. Information was gathered on age, education, sex, marital status, number of dependents, race, and whether the subject was a previous VR client. Those seven variables gathered from the case-service record were dichotomized; hence, there were 128 sets of characteristics a client could have. Applicants were assigned to one of the three outcome categories by use of a discrete discriminant function for classification of clients, embodying cost functions, which attempt to measure the costs of misclassifying a client.

Toms and Brewer then made assumptions on the relative magnitudes of the different costs of misclassification and demonstrated how a client would be assigned to a group depending on these cost assumptions. They then took a random sample of 18 clients—six from each group—and examined the performance of their discrete discrimination under different cost assumptions. The function seemed to have potential for use; however, the experiment should be replicated. The authors noted that the technique is "free of the usual normality, linearity, and homogeneity of variance assumptions inherent in most prediction procedures" (p. 237).

The research is mindful of loss functions in decision making under uncertainty. It also is similar in intent to integrated probability-benefit-cost research. While the introduction of the technique would not be difficult, potential users should exercise care to ensure that their sample sizes are relatively large. The need for a larger sample size is, perhaps, the main drawback of the scheme. If a researcher wanted to use 15 variables (not an uncommon situation in prediction research), there would be 32,768 possible sets of characteristics. Even with a sample size as large as 60,000 there would probably be empty cells. An applicant for services who had a set of characteristics that was empty in the sample could still be assigned, however, to a group on the basis of the frequency distribution of the three groups.

Brooks and Weaver, 1965

To determine whether psychomotor tests are valid predictors of release of psychiatric patients, the investigators chose Vermont State Hospital (2,175 population) as a site at which to administer five tests: reaction time, tapping rate, transport, assembly, and serial-reaction time. After excluding all those over 60 years old (reason given above), as well as the alcoholics and psychoneurotics (they had a high rate of release) and others for miscellaneous reasons, 1,203 observations were available.

The outcome measure was released within a one-year period. A two-way repeated measures ANOVA (outcome × Subject × Days) was applied. The in/out main effect was significant in 20 of 25 cases, and the five insignificant cases were all for the mentally deficient (see pp. 4.1, 4.4). In order to exploit that finding the authors used as observations in their multiple regression the correlation coefficients for age, sex, and five test scores with the criterion. The schizophrenic group (N = 636) was arrayed by age and every other observation was assigned to a validation group. The weights from that normative group were used to test the congruence between prediction and outcome (p. 4.5). Weights were also obtained for the entire sample, and predictions made on the subsamples.

The percentage of correct predictions was consistently high, ranging from 75 to 90 percent for the different diagnoses using own group weights, and from 74 to 86 percent for whole group weights.

The research screened out some of the initial population, generated some negative probability estimates and some greater than one (see p. 4.11), but it has great potential policy utility. The summary of usage potential in the SRS abstract (RD-1291) is on target:

1. It permits the use of a simple administered battery of performance tasks that may be given to all but the most regressed psychiatric patients.
2. Its avoidance of intellectual tasks allows it to be used by illiterate subjects.
3. The prediction scores available may be employed to determine the probability of rehabilitation success of psychiatric patients prior to the investment of considerable effort and expense.
4. There are indications that performance tasks are more responsive to changes in pathology of patients than more traditional psychological test measures.

The research has been partially replicated (see Burstein et al., 1967).

Peck and Stephens, 1964

This methodologically rich study is rather long and complex. We shall therefore simply attempt to transmit some of the flavor of the work.

In order to test four major hypotheses five random samples were used. Four of those were experimental and were drawn from different special-training situations for the mentally retarded; the fifth was a control group of retardates who attended the public schools. The hypotheses amalgamated as follows: a) the multitude of variables posited as related to rehabilitation success can be represented by factors that, in turn, will be significantly related to the success criterion (personal, sociocivic, and vocational success), and b) there will be differences in the success levels of those who received special training (higher) and those who did not (lower), as well as among the different groups.

The success criteria were represented by 141 variables—60 of those being 5-point ratings; 20 being continuous variables; and 61, dichotomies. There were 85 prediction variables, including eight dichotomies. All continuous variables were standardized, and <u>all</u> variables were normalized. Factor analysis resulted in the extraction of 17 criteria factors and 21 prediction factors. Multiple regression was run on the criteria (factor scores separately), with the 21 prediction factors as regressions. Fixed-effect models were used where the criteria or prediction set was composed of factor score and dichotomies or of dichotomy and factor score. ANOVA was employed to test the differences among groups hypothesis.

The conclusions and implications section of this study is 24-pages long. Its message is that the four hypotheses are accepted; that the predictions could be used to screen applicants for training; that the work should be replicated with a larger sample; that it be replicated over time; and that future designs include comparisons with the success of adult male normals.

Hoffman, 1969

A population of 569 patients discharged from Pineland Hospital and Training Center, Pownal, Maine, between July 1, 1952, and June 30, 1961, comprised the subjects for this study. Only nine of the discharged patients were lost to the study because they could not be located. Pre- and postdischarge information was available in the remaining 98 percent (560) of the population—an outstanding retention rate.

Four objective variables were chosen as criteria: the absence of police contacts, higher wage levels, full self-support, and domiciliary stability. Those were dichotomized, and a stepwise regression was run with 126 predischarge variables on the criteria. The sets selected in the multiple stepwise regression were used in discriminant function models (the IBM Scientific Subroutine Package version was used). The technique allowed for approximately 75-percent effectiveness of prediction. Different variables were selected, depending on the criterion, but the model usually contained only eight to ten variables.

The investigation lists the variables and the discriminant-function coefficients. It would be possible to cross validate, using the reported coefficients and a new sample. It would also be possible to alert counselors to recently-discharged retardates who need intensive assistance. An example might be that a client with a predicted likelihood of police contact could be given additional services to aid in his adjustment.

RECOMMENDATIONS

Strong consideration should be given to a series of pilot projects. One of those should accept all applicants for vocational rehabilitation. This could be done by having each federal-state agency in the nation accept 100 clients at random from the rehabilitation queue, without regard to counselor determination (counselors' evaluations could be made known for the record only). The sample of clients should proceed through the rehabilitation process in the usual fashion. Care should be taken to secure accurate information on the sample; multivariate statistical models should be utilized to choose the method that predicts outcomes with the highest degree of precision. The accuracy of the prediction should be checked with the recorded counselors' evaluations to determine the advantage—or lack of it—in the use of the statistical method. When such research is completed, it will give us a sample that is free from counselor selection bias and will enable us to investigate the possibility of statistical selection of clients, of rehabilitation as an entitlement, and so forth. In order to insure the cooperation of the state agencies in this project the government should agree to fund the incremental clients.

The second pilot project should apply statistical predictions on a prospective basis, thereby providing the acid test for the predictive technique.

It might be worthwhile to consider an alternative strategy that enables us to eliminate one of the pilot projects. We may estimate the coefficients of a statistical prediction model by applying it to data from the R-300 tapes.* Although the sample would be subject

---

*The computer files contain the case service record of rehabilitation clients and are gathered annually on a fiscal year basis.

to the bias of counselor presecreening as discussed above, we may
justify it on the grounds that the time and cost savings of elimination
of the first pilot project would be substantial, relative to the loss of
efficiency by this "second-best" approach. It that strategy were
adopted, the coefficients estimated could be applied immediately to
a randomly admitted sample of clients and the predictive power of the
statistical forecast compared with that of counselors.

If the projects described are undertaken, there is one obvious
obstacle that must be overcome. Those clients who were predicted
as failures by the counselors will be dealing with those very counselors
who saw them as unfit for the program. Counselors must therefore
not allow their own attitudes or behavior to affect the opportunity of
the group adversely. It will be difficult to develop a design that
guards against that threat.

If we are to sponsor research on the prediction of outcomes,
we should insist that the research design call for multidimensional
analysis and cross validation; univariate approaches are less likely
to bear fruit.

We should sponsor at least one national project that employs
the most productive design and techniques. Unfortunately, we do not
have an existing study done on a national sample, and we obviously
do not have one that has been validated over time.

If we can forecast outcome with 10 percent more accuracy than
we are doing now, both the savings in costs and the benefits to clients
and society would be substantial.

REFERENCES

A complete list of all the reports used in the preparation of
this chapter is available through the Disability and Health Economics
Research Section.

Bellante, D. M. "A Multivariate Analysis of a Vocational Rehabilita-
    tion Program." The Journal of Human Resources 7 (1972):
    226-41.

Bolton, B. "Predicting Client Outcome from Intake Data." Reha-
    bilitation Research and Practice Review 4 (1972): 23-26.

Brooks, G. W., and Weaver, L. A., Jr. Psychomotor Performance,
    Mental Disability and Rehabilitation. Burlington: University
    of Vermont, 1965.

Burstein, A.G., Soloff, A., Gillespie, H.G., and Haase, M. "Prediction of Hospital Discharge of Mental Patients by Psychomotor Performance: Partial Replication of Brooks and Weaver." Perceptual and Motor Skills 24 (1967): 127-34.

Campbell, D.T., and Stanley, J.C. Experimental and Quasi-Experimental Designs for Research. Chicago: Rand McNally, 1966.

Cobb, H.V. The Forecast of Fulfillment. New York: Teachers College Press, 1972.

Day, D., Cummings, R.J., Anderson, L.M., and Iverson, I.A. "Client Characteristics and Their Relation to Outcome: A Review of Previous Research." Mimeographed. Minnesota Institute of Interdisciplinary Studies, American Rehabilitation Foundation, Minneapolis, Minn., 1969.

De Mann, M.M. "A Predictive Study of Rehabilitation Counseling Outcomes." Journal of Counseling Psychology 10 (1963): 340-43.

Gilbert, D.H., and Lester, J.T. "The Relationships of Certain Personality and Demographic Variables to Success in Vocational Rehabilitation." Research Report from the Orthopedic Hospital, Los Angeles, Calif., 1970.

Goldberger, A.S. Econometric Theory. New York: Wiley, 1964.

Grigg, C.M., Holtman, A.G., and Martin, P.Y. Vocational Rehabilitation for the Disadvantaged. Lexington, Mass. Heath, 1970.

Hammond, C.D., Wright, G.N., and Butler, A.J. Caseload Feasibility in an Expanded Vocational Rehabilitation Program. The Wisconsin Studies in Vocational Rehabilitation, Series 2, Monograph VI. Madison, Wis.: University of Wisconsin, 1968.

Hoffman, T.L. An Investigation of Factors Contributing to Successful and Non-Successful Adjustment of Discharged Retardates. Pownal, Me.: The Pineland Hospital and Training Center, 1969.

Lenhart, L., Westerheide, W.J., Cowan, J.A., and Miller, M.C., III. "Description of Service Outcome Measurement Project: Two Approaches to Measuring Case Difficulty and Client Change." Rehabilitation Research and Practice Review 4 (1972): 27-33.

McNemar, Q. Psychological Statistics. 4th ed. New York: Wiley,
    1969.

Miller, L.A., and Allen, G. "The Prediction of Future Outcomes
    Among OASI Referrals Using NMZ Scores." Personnel and
    Guidance Journal 45 (1966): 349-52.

Morrison, D.G. "Upper Bounds for Correlations Between Binary
    Outcomes and Probabilistic Predictions." Journal of the
    American Statistical Association 67 (1972): 68-70.

Nerlove, M., and Press, S.J. Univariate and Multivariate Log-
    linear and Logistic Models. Santa Monica, Calif.: The Rand
    Corp., 1973.

Neter, J., and Maynes, E.S. "On the Appropriateness of the Corre-
    lation Coefficient with a 0, 1 Dependent Variable." Journal
    of the American Statistical Association 65 (1970): 501-09.

Noble, J.H., Jr. "Actuarial System for Weighting Case Closures."
    Rehabilitation Record 14, no. 5 (September-October 1973):
    34-37.

Novis, F. W., Marra, J.L., and Zadrozny, L.J. "Qualitative
    Measurement in the Initial Screening of Rehabilitation Potential."
    Personnel and Guidance Journal 39 (1960): 262-69.

Peck, J.R., and Stephens, W.B. Success of Young Male Retardates.
    Austin, Tex.: The University of Texas, 1964.

Reagles, K.W., Wright, G.N., and Butler, A.J. Correlates of
    Client Satisfaction in an Expanded Vocational Rehabilitation
    Program. The Wisconsin Studies in Vocational Rehabilitation,
    Monograph XII. Madison, Wis.: University of Wisconsin,
    1970a.

________. A Scale of Rehabilitation Gain for Clients of an Expanded
    Vocational Rehabilitation Program. The Wisconsin Studies in
    Vocational Rehabilitation, Monograph XIII. Madison, Wis.:
    University of Wisconsin, 1970b.

Rubin, S.E., Bolton, B., and Salley, K. A Review of the Literature
    on the Prediction of Rehabilitation Client Outcome and the
    Development of a Research Model. Arkansas Studies in

Vocational Rehabilitation, Monograph V. Fayetteville, Ark.:
Arkansas Rehabilitation Research and Training Center, 1973.

Rubin, S.E., and Salley, K. Studies of Prediction of Rehabilitation
Outcome: An Annotated Bibliography. Fayetteville, Ark.: The
Arkansas Rehabilitation Research and Training Center, 1973.

Sawyer, J. "Measurement and Prediction, Clinical and Statistical."
Psychological Bulletin 66 (1966): 178-200.

Segal, S.P. "Research on the Outcome of Social Work Therapeutic
Interventions: A Review of the Literature." Journal of Health
and Social Behavior 13 (1972): 3-17.

Sinnett, E.R., Stimpert, W.E., Wilkins, D.M., and Straight, E.
A Five Year Follow-Up Study of Psychiatric Patients. Manhattan, Kans.: Kansas State University, 1965.

Stein, C.I., Bradley, A.D., and Buegel, B.L. "A Test of Basic
Assumptions Underlying Vocational Counseling Utilizing a
Differential Criterion Method." Journal of Counseling Psy-
chology 17 (1970): 93-97.

Toms, J.G., and Brewer, J.K. "A Discrete Discriminant Analysis
Procedure for Vocational Rehabilitation Predictions." Rehabilitation Literature 32 (1971): 232-38.

Tseng, M.S. "Predicting Vocational Rehabilitation Dropouts from
Psychometric Attributes and Work Behaviors." Rehabilitation
Counseling Bulletin 16 (1972): 154-59.

Westerheide, W.J., and Lenhart, L. Case Difficulty and Client
Change: A Review of the Literature. Monograph I. Oklahoma
City, Okla.: Oklahoma Department of Institutions, Social and
Rehabilitation Services, 1974.

______. "Development and Reliability of a Pretest-Posttest Rehabilita-
tion Services Outcome Measure." Rehabilitation Research and
Practice Review 4 (1973): 15-24.

12

REHABILITATION RESEARCH FOCUSING ON ORGANIZATIONAL VARIABLES

Rehabilitation is an interpersonal process but one which necessarily occurs in organizational settings designated "people-changing" by some sociologists (Hasenfeld and English, 1972, p. 5; Vinter, 1963). We will focus on two major categories of research: research examining "coordination of services" and research investigating rehabilitation settings for the "severely handicapped." The first refers to projects that examine the effectiveness of either an interorganizational arrangement for the processing of clients or a single-agency multiservice approach. We have examined 50 such projects. By the "severely handicapped" we mean those persons who have been defined, either a priori or on the basis of prior rehabilitation experience, as having low probabilities of being successfully rehabilitated. We have examined 22 projects of that type.

Since it may not be apparent why such projects are being considered as a category of research dealing with organizational issues related to rehabilitation, some explanation is in order. First of all, classification of clients (screening in or out) occurs systematically as an organizational activity. Decisions about the kinds of disabled persons who can or should be treated represent organizational policy. Even when they do not represent formal policy, decisions to screen out certain classes of handicapped persons are often traceable to the organizational phenomenon of "goal displacement." Moreover, once the status of "severely handicapped" has been conferred upon a

---

This chapter was written by Jack Oldham, Research Associate, Department of Sociology, Rutgers University, and Bernard Goldstein, Professor, Department of Sociology, Rutgers University.

disabled person, his or her case is presumed to pose a different sort of challenge, for which a different sort of organizational response is required.

RESEARCH ON COORDINATION OF REHABILITATIVE SERVICES

The 50 research projects reviewed under the heading of "coordination of services" are difficult to further categorize in terms of their subject matter. Forty percent (N = 20) of these studies investigated coordination of rehabilitative services for the mentally retarded and mentally ill; 14 percent (N = 7) focused on the distribution of services to the educationally and socially disadvantaged. The remaining studies, just less than half the total (N = 23), were distributed across a variety of substantive areas, including programs for alcoholics, public offenders, the aged, and persons with orthopedic or sensory handicaps. In most cases, the projects were intended to assess the extent to which new and/or improved services could be offered to clientele through an alteration or innovation in organizational arrangements for the delivery of services. In some cases, the object was the inclusion of a new or different sort of clientele within the population eligible for rehabilitation. Programs or plans of service ordinarily included cooperation among various agencies or innovative approaches to coordinated services by subcomponents within a single agency. Early identification of clients, the use of existing community agencies as referral sources, altered or improved screening processes, relocation of the loci of control and coordination, and similar measures comprised the nature of the innovation in most cases.

The majority (76 percent) of the research was conducted by institutions or agencies that are ordinarily engaged in rehabilitation on a regular basis: 38 percent (N = 19) by state vocational-rehabilitation agencies, 24 percent (N = 12) by private rehabilitation agencies, and 14 percent (N = 7) by other state agencies (e.g., corrections, health, and so on.) involved in rehabilitative programs. Thus, it is not surprising to find that the research might almost invariably be classified as "self-evaluation" conducted by personnel involved in the programs being evaluated (84 percent; N = 42). Only 6 percent (N = 3) of the studies were conducted by independent third parties. Most, of course, were "project reports," the traditional form of self-evaluation effort.

Research Technique

Some observations are in order before proceeding to question
the methodological adequacy of the studies. It should be acknowledged
that much of the research analyzed here represents routine project
reports of demonstration projects of various kinds. Thus, as will
become evident below, relatively little attention has been given to
control groups, randomization of sampling, and so forth. Most of
the studies are case studies, naturally, rather than comparative
assessments.

But to regard such approaches as understandable in their context is not to condone them as appropriate research orientations.
Randomization of cases, admittedly, is difficult to justify in programs
that exist to provide services. Assignment of cases to control groups
may lead to charges of "denial of services." Self-selection tendencies
and practitioners' proclivities to assign the "most deserving" cases
to experimental treatment groups are common occurrences that are
often difficult to condemn. Yet they detract from the quality and
utility of research (Freeman and Sherwood, 1965).

While almost two-thirds (N = 31) of the studies were classifiable
as either experimental or "quasi-experimental" designs (Campbell
and Stanley, 1966), only 16 percent (N = 8) employed control groups
of any sort. One-third (N = 16) were "one-shot case studies"; many
of them were demonstration projects. There were also 16 other
demonstration projects that were nonexperimental under even the
broadly inclusive category of "quasi-experimental" designs employed
here.

Attention paid to sampling procedures seems to be another
reasonable indicant of the general research orientations employed in
the studies. More than three-quarters of the 50 studies (N = 38)
cannot be considered to be based on a "sample" in any formal sense.
Only five studies employed randomization techniques. For the most
part, cases exposed to the innovative treatment were selected on a
first-come-first-served basis, but self-selection and professional
referrals of selected clients for this sort of "special" treatment
clearly played roles in determining the composition of the "samples."
It should also be acknowledged that, to the extent that that also typifies
the ways in which clients find their ways into ordinary programs,
critics ought to look beyond sampling procedures to assess the worth
of the programs. In any event, from the research standpoint, laxity
with respect to sampling is hardly encouraging.

Quality research relies upon strong analytical techniques for
making inferences and evaluating hypotheses. Table 12.1 illustrates
the extent to which the research projects relied upon certain kinds of

TABLE 12.1

Statistical Analyses Employed in 50 Reports Dealing
with Coordination of Services

Analysis	Number	Percent
Simple descriptive techniques (mostly percentages, tables, means)	46	92
Associational analysis (mostly Chi-square tests)	14	28
Simple correlational analysis	5	10
Analysis of variance and covariance	3	6
Regression analysis	1	2
Factor analysis	0	0

Note: Percentages add up to more than 100 percent, because some projects employed more than one of the above techniques.

statistical analyses in testing their hypotheses and presenting their conclusions. It is clear that there is a strong inverse relationship between the discriminative power of a technique and the likelihood of its having been employed in the research analyzed.

That relationship is most discouraging when one considers that one of the most important questions concerning any rehabilitation program is not merely whether it can be made to work but the conditions under which it will work. It is difficult to imagine how this question can be adequately answered on the basis of descriptive statistics alone. Yet this was the predominant pattern in the reports.

Thus, to evaluate the 50 reports in terms of their general research orientations as indicated by the research designs utilized, the attention paid to sampling, and the statistical techniques employed, is to conclude that they have serious shortcomings.

Indicants of Research Rigor

An examination of some more subtle indicants of the rigor with which such research has been conducted yields equally disappointing findings.

Nearly all the research examined programs in terms of the outcomes in the cases of participating clients. Thus, one would assume that interpretation of findings would depend in part upon the effects upon the case-mix of nonresponses, referrals, and program dropouts. Yet the research overwhelmingly neglected to provide such information or to take it into account in the analysis if it was provided. Sixty-eight percent (N = 34) of the reports examined furnished no information as to nonresponses. Only three projects adjusted their statistical analysis to accommodate nonresponse rates. Seventy-six percent (N = 38) of projects failed to mention how "refusals" (persons declining to participate) may have influenced either the composition of the sample or the computation of success rates. Although 13 reports showed that "dropouts" either did not occur or had been taken into account in the analysis, the majority of the reports (72 percent; N = 36) did not acknowledge the dropout problem or, if they did so, failed to adjust for it in the analysis.

All the standard texts on evaluation research emphasize the importance of defining program goals explicitly so that resultant hypotheses can be clearcut and testable. Yet in 16 of the studies (32 percent) the raters could not identify the hypotheses, even though they had been instructed to "read into" the research objectives more than was explicitly stated. Among those studies whose hypotheses were spelled out an additional 30 percent (N = 15) were rated as being nontestable or overly vague, and so on. Thus, in almost two-thirds of the research projects (N = 31) the hypotheses could not be ascertained or were severely flawed in terms of their utility in drawing conclusions.

It also seems important that researchers consider alternative or rival hypotheses for their findings. Yet only 11 of the studies (22 percent) recognized and stated at least one alternative explanation for their findings, and only eight (16 percent) actually explored the alternatives through analysis of the data. That finding is of course quite consonant with the observation above, that the great majority of the reports utilized only descriptive statistics, thus making exploration of rival hypotheses all but impossible in most cases.

Follow-Up Studies

A subtle but extremely important measure of program effectiveness is the duration of the client's exposure to a treatment program. In the majority of the research examined, however, that factor was neither carefully measured as a case variable nor controlled in the analysis. Thus, if two clients entered a program in which one lasted for two weeks, the other for two months, they were not ordinarily distinguished from each other on that basis in the analysis. Both would have been considered "exposed"; no measure of degree of exposure was typically controlled for in the analysis. Half the reports (N = 25) presumably could have conducted such analysis, as they were able to provide average exposure figures for all clients, but failed to subdivide clients into groups on that basis. Since length of treatment, on even an intuitive basis, would appear to be a most important variable for consideration in such studies, its omission in most studies must be regarded as a significant negative finding. Many programs may have "threshold effects" such that rehabilitation of a client is not a reasonable expectation until the client has spent X units of time in the program or had received X units of contact with program features. Such information is typically not provided.

Serious consideration of rehabilitation outcomes, especially when "success" is operationally defined as employed status at a given point in time, would seem to call for considerable attention to follow-up studies. Treatment periods ranged from less than one month to over two years in the studies, with the modal collapsed category being three to 12 months (N = 14; 28 percent). One-fifth of the studies conducted true follow-ups—that is, efforts to learn about the status of former clients at a point in time beyond the normal end of the clients' participation in the program. Eight studies suggested or proposed follow-ups but, for various reasons, did not conduct them. Sixty-four percent (N = 32) of the reports made no mention of follow-ups in the sense that the term is used here. This may be due more to the absence of funding for follow-up studies than to any systematic lack of concern on the part of researchers. However, since the final determination of "closed rehabilitated" or some other status often takes place at, or very close to the time of release or placement of clients, there is considerable risk of the Hawthorne effect influencing the findings, often artificially inflating the true or lasting success rate. Since only 26 percent (N = 13) of the projects examined were considered to have been conducted by the "regular crew" of the institutions, there also would seem to be an attendant risk of a halo effect due to special conditions in the internal environment of these programs. Where such conditions are a factor, considerably more attention to follow-up studies seems warranted.

Controlling for Conditions That Attend Upon Results

From the sociological perspective, as mentioned above, it is extremely important to note the conditions under which organizational innovations seem to "work." Some innovations can be expected to differentially succeed due to individual differences in clients' past experiences or statuses and/or in the socioeconomic conditions that characterize their backgrounds or the environment. To be useful, therefore, research on rehabilitation should document those conditions. Then subsequent programs can be planned in the knowledge of the effects of client-related or situational variables, some of which may serve as good predictors of program outcomes. Unfortunately, scant attention has been paid to controlling for the conditions that attend the results obtained in the reports.

While the average report recorded between six and nine variables related to clients (mean equals 8.2; median equals 6.5), most reports utilized such information only to <u>describe</u> clients. Relatively few reports seriously attempted to document relevant relationships among variables that intervene in the rehabilitation process. Virtually none did so in any sophisticated manner, such as the utilization of multiple treatment groups and/or the application of multivariate techniques in the statistical analysis.

Methodology Ratings

The preceding sections have contained many negative findings about the ways in which research on coordination of rehabilitation services has typically been done. If the 50 projects are at all typical of the universe of such research, some very serious questions must be raised about the methodological adequacy of studies in this field. Eighty-six percent (N = 43) of the reports were rated on the lower half of the scale of methodological adequacy (five or below). In fact, exactly half of them received minimal scores (one or two points). The entire distribution of the scores was heavily skewed toward the negative end of the rating scale (mean equals 3.4; median equals 2.0; mode equals 2.0).*

---

*Because the subjective ratings were so low (and because a few projects in the other subsample were rated by a different person), another rating scale was constructed on the basis of more objective criteria from the checklist. Scores on that 9-point scale ranged from one to seven. Eighty-six percent (N = 43) once again scored five points or less. While those scores were slightly higher than the subjective ratings, they nonetheless clustered on the lower half of the scale (mean equals 4.08; median equals 4.0; mode equals 3.0). Each study received one point for each of the following: (a) if checklister recorded no doubts as to generalizability based upon sampling, (b) if

Research Outcomes

In a book on the methods of evaluation research Carol Weiss asserts that there has been a tendency on the part of evaluators to conclude that programs have had "little effect" (1972, pp. 126-28). Such findings jeopardize the existence and continuation of programs. We wish to stress, therefore, that we have reviewed research on rehabilitation programs—not the programs themselves. While our findings may suggest that research is largely ineffective, they should not be construed as criticisms of the programs that such research examines.

For the most part, the research that we reviewed on coordination of rehabilitation services did not conclude that programs had little effect. In fact, fully 92 percent (N = 46) of these fifty studies reported that their major hypotheses had found support (i.e., could not be rejected). Those hypotheses usually stated that the introduction of innovations a, b, and c would produce changes x, y, and z that, in turn, constituted "improved" services. Such findings, in effect, show overwhelmingly that the programs resulted in improvements upon the status quo in rehabilitation.

As shown above, those favorable conclusions rest upon very questionable methodological grounds. There are phenomena and relationships, it is true, that are so striking that they will become apparent under even the most shoddy research conditions. Yet we must agree with Weiss that such cases are the exceptions rather than the rule, and that it is more realistic to expect evaluation studies to show "small, ambiguous changes, minor effects, outcomes influenced by specific events of the place and the moment" (Weiss, 1972 p. 3). Thus, it is difficult for us to accept the notion that the laxity that permits researchers to utilize such poor methodologies suddenly gives way to rigor in the area of conclusions about hypotheses. Rather, we must be suspicious of such overwhelmingly optimistic research findings, because they are based upon the weak methodological grounds found here.

We reiterate that many of the programs themselves may be exemplary. We cannot conclude, however, that we have learned much

---

data sources were rated sufficient, (c) if the design was experimental or at least quasi-experimental, (d) if hypotheses were adequately spelled out, (e) if rival hypotheses were at least acknowledged, (f) if descriptive statistics were used, (g) if associational analysis was employed, (h) if correlational analysis was employed, and (i) if multivariate techniques were employed in the analysis.

about such programs or the conditions under which they succeed <u>on</u>
<u>the basis of most of the fifty research reports examined here</u>.

In light of our findings with respect to their methodology, it
should not be surprising that these research reports received poor
ratings in terms of their "policy utility." Projects received favorable
ratings on this scale to the extent that they were characterized by
one or more of the following conditions:

- Findings were of sufficient importance to warrant replication of
  the project and the evaluation.
- Findings were judged to be reliable support to on-going policy.
- Findings, even if not completely reliable, strongly suggest the
  need to reexamine existing policy.

Seventy percent (N = 35) of the studies scored five points or
less on the ten-point policy-utility scale. The distribution of scores
approximated a normal curve somewhat more closely than did either
of the methodology scales, but nonetheless it was skewed toward the
lower end of the scale (mean equals 4.3; median equals 4.0; mode
equals 1.5). Twelve studies (24 percent), however did score seven
or more points on the scale, which is indicative of contributions to
our knowledge about rehabilitation.

Of particular interest with respect to policy utility are three
studies that achieved rather high ratings. Dibner et al. demonstrated,
through the utilization of a control-group design, that improved rehabilitative services could be offered to aged welfare clients by means
of interagency collaboration between welfare and public rehabilitation
agencies. A study by Educational Evaluation and Research Associates
focused on cases in a similar interagency arrangement and employed
sophisticated statistical analyses for the achievement of a predictive
model, based on a variety of socioeconomic variables, of the rehabilitation outcomes of low-income males. The same organizational
arrangement was examined by Pagan (1968) in his pretest/posttest
study of welfare clients eligible for rehabilitation in a district of
Puerto Rico. The net effect of those studies has been to suggest that
welfare and rehabilitation programs can cooperate effectively in
providing services to disabled clients. Such cooperation may prove
beneficial to the community as well by removing clients from the
welfare rolls.

While it is difficult to attribute to any one reason the poor
ratings in policy utility earned by the remainder of the studies, we
must point out that an exceptionally strong correlation existed between
scores on the methodology (subjective) scale and policy-utility ratings
$(r = .82; p \leq .001)$. In other words, poor methodology was a prime
detractor from the generalizability—and, therefore, usefulness—of
many of the studies examined.

TABLE 12.2

Levels of Contributions to Knowledge of Rehabilitation
of 50 Research Reports on Coordination
of Rehabilitation Services

Contribution	Number	Percent
Practical application of techniques	31	62
Empirical findings	16	32
Conceptual contributions	13	26

Note: Percentages do not add up to 100 percent, because
some projects made more than one sort of contribution. Five
reports were rated as making none of the contributions.

Closely related to the question of policy utility is the nature
of the contribution that each research project sought to make to our
knowledge of the rehabilitation process. Table 12.2 shows the distribution among research projects in terms of the levels of their
contributions. It is interesting to note that the higher the level of
contribution, the smaller the proportion of reports classified as
having made such contributions.

True conceptual developments are relatively rare byproducts
of research done largely as self-evaluation by program practitioners,
as the majority of this research was done. Bernstein et al. (1973,
pp. 108ff.) have theorized that the "major audience" to which reports
are addressed (i.e., one's reference group) is a good predictor of
adherence to scientific norms. A theoretical-conceptual orientation
to the research is one such norm. Most of the reports we considered
were written by practitioners either for other practitioners or for
funding agencies. Thus, the lack of concern with conceptual contributions is neither surprising nor particularly disturbing.

Ordinarily, we might prefer findings that purport to contribute
to our knowledge of practical applications of techniques and/or empirical tests of existing rehabilitation models. But such findings
typically contribute little unless they teach us something about the
various conditions under which such techniques can be successfully
implemented. In these reports, the absence of control groups and
the inattention to control for even those variables that were recognized
made such contributions largely impossible.

To summarize, the returns on the investment in rehabilitation
research on coordination of services have been disappointing; such
research clearly has more potential. Little has been learned, in

comparison to what could have been learned. With a few notable exceptions, little credible evidence has been generated that sheds light in a systematic way upon the question of "what works" in the coordination of rehabilitative services. Many good opportunities to answer important questions have evidently been lost. The major reason for the lack of useful findings is inadequate or marginally adequate methodology. Some, but not all, of the methodological shortcomings can be attributed to researchers' making the best of a difficult research situation. We might better seek explanations for the majority of the problems, however, in the role conflicts that face practitioners doing research in settings where the overriding organizational commitments are to service rather than research.

RESEARCH ON THE REHABILITATION OF THE SEVERELY HANDICAPPED

Our findings with respect to research on the organization of rehabilitative services for the severely handicapped conform quite closely to the patterns cited above with respect to coordination of services. That is, we must express severe reservations, based primarily upon the poor methodological quality of most of the twenty-two reports examined, about what has been learned in this field. Because of the similarity between findings with respect to this group of studies and those already reported, the narrative will be minimized here.

The research projects evaluating rehabilitation specifically directed at severely handicapped persons present no particular pattern with regard to subject matter. Orthopedic handicaps were the focal points of six studies. Three concentrated upon sensory handicaps; two on mental retardation. The remaining half represented an assortment of areas. What most of the projects had in common was their definition of the target population of the program as "severely handicapped." That was operationally defined in terms of a group of clients who had either been screened out of previous programs or, if they had been accepted, had "failed" to be rehabilitated. Frequently, clients with multiple handicaps were the subjects of the program. Rediagnoses and special intensive-treatment programs typified those efforts.

Half the research examined in that category (N = 11) was conducted by private rehabilitation agencies. Five studies (23 percent) were done by universities and medical schools. The remaining six (27 percent) were done by state agencies, hospitals, and so forth. In 19 of the 22 cases (86 percent) the research was conducted by members of the staff of the project and represented "self-evaluation."

All twenty two projects were funded by SRS. The projects were
carried out from 1954 to 1972. The years 1959-64 saw the most
intense activity and accounted for more than half of the research
(N = 12).

Research Technique

Our examination of research techniques disclosed a number of
weaknesses comparable to those in the studies on coordination of
services.

Thirteen of the studies employed nonexperimental designs. Of
those studies that were experimental in the broadest sense (N = 19)
only one employed a control-group design of any kind. Six were
one-shot case studies. Most were conceived as demonstration projects
of some sort.

While most of the studies probably had enough cases for drawing
conclusions about techniques (50 percent; N = 11 had Ns $\geq$ 100),
relatively few engaged in any formal sampling procedures. In four-
fifths of the cases the "samples" were neither randomly nor systematically drawn. Ordinarily, the studies made the assumption that
cases were representative of the case mix that had been (or would
be) the norm for the organization. (The assumption was rarely
demonstrated.)

As in our earlier findings, we observed a tendency to rely
almost exclusively upon simple descriptive statistics in reaching
conclusions and communicating results in project reports. Table 12.3
shows that the same pattern existed: The greater the discriminatory
power of a technique, the less likely it was to have been employed.

Thus, on the basis of selection of research designs, attention
to sampling, and the sophistication of analytical techniques employed,
most of these studies invite considerable criticism.

Indicants of Research Rigor

When we analyze more subtle measures of the rigor that
characterized the research efforts, we find additional shortcomings.
Scant attention was paid to the handling of those phenomena of case
getting that may affect the interpretation of results: dropout, refusal,
and nonresponse rates. Only one report adjusted for the occurence
of dropouts. Seven others described the problem but did not take it
into account in the analysis. Twelve reports (55 percent) made no

TABLE 12.3

Statistical Analyses Employed in 22 Reports Dealing
with Rehabilitation Programs for the
Severely Handicapped

Analysis	Number	Percent
Simple descriptive techniques	20	91
Associational analysis	5	23
Simple correlational analysis	3	14
Analysis of variance and covariance	0	0
Regression analysis	0	0
Factor analysis	0	0

Note: Percentages add up to more than 100 percent, because some projects employed more than one of the techniques.

mention of dropouts. Coincidentally, 86 percent (N = 19) of the reports failed to provide any information on either the refusal or nonresponse rates or on the handling of same.

Two-fifths of the projects failed to spell out hypotheses or to provide any basis on which raters could extrapolate them. But among those that did, another six (27 percent) were rated as having short-comings in terms of being overly vague, nontestable, and so on. Thus, in two-thirds of the cases (N = 16) there were problems related to the crucial research step of spelling out hypotheses with sufficient clarity to permit their later rejection, if warranted. Nor were these projects particularly attentive to alternative hypotheses. Rival hypotheses were recognized in only five cases (23 percent), none of which ana-lyzed the data in that light.

In half the cases examined there is no mention of the duration of clients' exposure to the treatment variables, either as average (group) data or as a variable for each client. That has to be regarded as a significant deficiency.

None of the studies conducted a follow-up that was independent of the program design itself. Over half (N = 12) even neglected to record the duration of the interval between the end of treatment and the final measurement of change in the dependent variable. Thus, it is extremely difficult to draw upon the studies under consideration for any reliable assessment of the lasting impact of programs for the rehabilitation of the severely handicapped.

Controlling for Conditions That Attend upon Results

As in the case of research on the coordination of services, there is little attention paid in the group of reports under review to analyzing the conditions under which various results obtain. For example, of these 22 reports only three analyzed the effects of social class upon the rehabilitation process. Seventeen studies failed even to note clients' occupational histories, although "rehabilitation" almost by definition is appraised in occupational terms. Obviously, the question of prior occupational experience will not be relevant for all severely handicapped groups, as some will have had lifelong disabilities precluding work experience. But it seems reasonable that more than four projects could have analyzed for the effects upon rehabilitation outcomes of clients' past work experiences.

Summary indexes on the number of variables considered and the strength of the consideration each received are disappointing. While the typical report in the group recognized some eight to ten variables related to clients (mean equals 9.8; median equals 8.3; mode equals 8.0), it was rare indeed for those variables to be employed in anything more than a narrative fashion; although their role was acknowledged, it was neither explored nor analyzed. The "strength" of the treatment received by each variable averaged two points on the five-point scale (mean equals 2.0; median equals 2.0; mode equals 2.0). That is a minimal score associated with variables that were merely mentioned. Variables that were systematically recorded and displayed, even for purely descriptive purposes, received higher scores than the averages here.

Because of their inadequate control of client-related variables, the reports cannot enlighten us about the conditions that are associated with differential success rates in the rehabilitation of the severely handicapped.

Methodology Ratings

Summary indexes with respect to methodology are no more encouraging than the findings already discussed. The subjective ratings on seven of the 22 projects were done by another panelist whose ratings were typically higher than our own. Despite that fact, half the projects received minimal ratings in methodology (one or two points out of a possible ten), and almost two-thirds (N = 14) were rated on the lower half of the scale (mean equals 4.3; median equals 2.0; mode equals 2.0).

By the nine-point objective scale described in the section on the methodology of research on coordination of services, the projects also rated rather poorly. No project scored more than five points on the scale (mean equals 3.6; median equals 4.0; mode equals 4.0). Thus, the two measures corroborate one another once again. That suggests that the reports as a group can be characterized as poor in their methodology.

Research Outcomes

When one asks what has been learned on the basis of the group of reports, the answer is "comparatively little." Many of the reports were from demonstration projects. While their major research hypotheses were almost invariably supported (91 percent; $N = 20$), the question remains, of whether they <u>convincingly</u> demonstrated the efficacy of the programs.

Our conviction is that, while many of the programs that the research projects investigated may have been quite effective and advantageous from a variety of viewpoints, we would be reluctant to rely solely upon the testimony of the reports. A careful reading of the reports leaves the impression that useful and innovative programs have indeed been undertaken. But the goal of research is the generation of convincing and conclusive evidence, not merely the stimulation of favorable impressions.

Once again, it is possible to point to methodological flaws as the primary reasons for the low ratings given many reports with respect to policy utility. The correlation between the subjective measure of methodological adequacy and the policy-utility scale was extremely high ($r = .89$; $p \leq .001$). Forty-one percent ($N = 9$) received minimal ratings (one or two points) on the ten-point policy-utility scale. While one-third ($N = 7$) of the reports were rated at the top of the scale (nine or ten points), those were primarily reports rated by another panelist whose ratings considerable exceeded our own. While the average report was rated as moderately important in terms of its contributions to policy making (mean equals 5.4; median equals 5.0; mode equals 2.0), that figure must be regarded at least in part as the product of idiosyncratic evaluations.

Eight projects in this group (36 percent) were rated by check-listers as having made no contribution to our knowledge of rehabilitation. Three sought to make conceptual contributions. Four aimed at empirical documentation of some rehabilitation or organization model for service. And seven sought to demonstrate that procedures could be effectively put into practice.

We do not argue that the group of reports failed to demonstrate anything of substance. Some reports did succeed in meeting their objectives and in making significant contributions. Two studies in particular merit discussion because they rated high on both methodology and policy-utility scales. A descriptive study by Roth and Eddy (1967) focused on the rehabilitation of disadvantaged clients in a city public hospital. It is commendable for its attention to the difficulties related to institutional depersonalization and role conflicts among actors in the rehabilitation setting. The study identified the social and economic factors that differentiated between successful and failing rehabilitation clients. Major weaknesses were found in the process itself: accidental and arbitrary admissions patterns, no arrangement for transition of clients out of total care modality, and staff roles that stressed custodial over therapeutic factors.

Sharples and Crawford (1972) followed the behavior of child amputees for an extended period beyond the treatment process. They examined the influence on both social and physical rehabilitation outcomes of numerous "social performance" factors, such as parental expectations and levels of participation in various peer activities. They also analyzed—indeed, controlled for—the effects of numerous demographic variables as well as physical characteristics of the disability. The result is an exceedingly useful inventory of the conditions that account for more favorable adjustment of childhood amputees.

The pessimism that has characterized our assessments of the majority of the research on the organization of services for the severely handicapped is perhaps better understood when our appraisals are set in a relative context. That is, we cannot help being critical of the general quality of the research examined here, in view of the largely unfulfilled potential such research appears to have offered at one time. Had more of these studies lived up to their potential, we might know a great deal more than we do of the process of rehabilitating the severely handicapped and the conditions under which such efforts succeed. Collectively, the reports frustrate the social scientist who sees evaluation research as a potentially significant tool assisting decision makers in their efforts to allocate resources on a more rational basis.

SUMMARY AND CONCLUSIONS

The rehabilitation research that examines organizational issues typically excludes both rigorous collection of data on socioeconomic variables and careful analysis of the effects of such variables on rehabilitation. Safilios-Rothschild, in her review of rehabilitation research findings, identified 36 factors that have been shown in one or more studies to be significantly related to the client's "post-disability gainful employment" (1970, pp. 230-35). It is particularly regrettable that those are so infrequently considered in studies of the organizational context of rehabilitation. Any effort to utilize such information in order to achieve more favorable outcomes would require translation into bureaucratic structure.

For example, the disabled person's perceptions of the attitudes of "significant others" toward disability clearly intervene in the rehabilitation process. Efforts to ameliorate the situation, such as family therapy programs, require organizational implementation. Yet most of the organizational research on rehabilitation ignores mediating variables, thus precluding <u>informed</u> efforts to control for their effects in later programs.

A variety of suggestions come to mind for improving the quality of research. They derive from our interpretation of the data and impressions of what can and cannot be found in the research reports examined.

First, we urge that a clear distinction be made in the future between "project reports" and "program evaluations." We recognize that the reports reviewed here have not all been written for the same reason and that it is not necessarily fair to apply criteria for judging research quality to documents intended to fulfill another purpose entirely. In reading the reports, one gets the impression that many were written not primarily to communicate research findings, but rather in satisfaction of requirements for evidence that programs have been carried out and monitored. Such "research" must be regarded as tangential to the ordinary responsibilities and interests of rehabilitation practitioners. Those responsible quite correctly view their primary roles as running programs for the delivery of rehabilitation services and structure their priorities, budget, time, and personal resources accordingly. Under those conditions, the temporary merger of the researcher and practitioner roles results in the resolution of role and time conflicts at the expense of research responsibilities. Several authors have noted the incompatibility of the research and practitioner roles in organizational settings (Arsonson and Sherwood, 1967; Argyris, 1958; Pelz, 1956). Perhaps the principal explanation for the poor quality of the research is to be sought in that phenomenon.

It may be that in certain situations funding agencies are completely satisfied to receive "project reports" that, whatever their quality, attest to the fact that a funded program has in fact been completed and that some attention has been paid to thoughtful interpretation of results. At other times, however, agencies may prefer a research project that is generalizable with regard to policy, and in which all results are thoroughly explored. The problem here has been that the term "research" has not been restricted to the latter type of study.

It is conceivable that the poor quality of the research is also due in part to low expectations on the part of the funding agency or failure to communicate the level of expectations that do apply. If that is true, the situation is not nearly as hopeless as it might otherwise appear. An important first step in its remediation might be the adoption by funding agencies of policies to facilitate communication about the appropriate content of research reports. Other conclusions have been drawn that relate to the role of the funding agency in the social control of research and to the location of the evaluation component vis-a-vis the program. (Chapter 14 has a fuller discussion of these and related issues.)

Practitioners are in some respects advantageously placed to make contributions of certain kinds. In cases where project personnel _are_ doing the research there is the opportunity to record systematically first-person accounts of the problems that inhere in the running of rehabilitation programs. The present reward system, however, actually discourages practitioners from including such information. Instead, they are led to adopt the guise of the impartial observer and to suppress any information that indicates that they also ran the program. Again, that is a problem that derives from the intrarole conflicts often forced upon practitioners who, when it is time to write up program results, don their "researcher" garments. That can be counterproductive, because there is a need for precisely the sorts of "operations" information that is so often purged from reports. A more extensive body of literature in this regard would prove immensely valuable by adding to our understanding of the organizational context of rehabilitation.

Specific recommendations emerged with respect to avenues of referral into the rehabilitation "stream" and the consequences of the reification of arbitrary eligibility criteria in our legal structure. (A discussion of these and related issues is contained in Chapter 15.)

Some specific observations are in order with respect to the areas that the reports on rehabilitation research on organizational variables did not address but that seem to require research.

Our review of research on the rehabilitation of the severely handicapped suggests that many persons previously considered high failure risks can in fact be rehabilitated. There is great need for research on the costs and consequences of diagnostic procedures that become routinized at levels that, while they suffice for modal client groups, are not sufficiently sensitive to identify the rehabilitation potential of severely handicapped clients.

It should also be kept in mind that people-processing organizations in general rely extensively upon classification and labelling procedures for the initial disposition of clients' cases: "From a sociological perspective, the important thing about any diagnosis, whether correctly established or not, is that it involves questions of definition" (Glaser and Strauss, 1968, p. 8). The diagnosis stage is important from the organizational point of view as a mechanism that sorts cases into convenient pigeonholds. From the client's perspective that phase of the career is important for reasons of socialization: That is the point at which he or she learns to accept or deal with a new or reaffirmed definition of self.

Initial classifications in turn create instances of the "self-fulfilling prophecy," in which clients learn to behave in accordance with their diagnoses, ultimately affirming the "truth" of the applied labels. That has been shown to be the case with respect to the "Pygmalion effect" in school classrooms (Rosenthal and Jacobson, 1968), the socialization of blind persons into dependency roles (Scott, 1969, Ch. 2), the institutionalization of mental patients (Rosenhan, 1973), prisoner-guard relationships (Zimbardo, 1973), the treatment of hospital emergency-room patients (Roth, 1972), and even the behavior of dying patients and those with whom they interact (Glaser and Strauss, 1968). The client's fate in many cases is at least as much a function of the diagnosis as of any intrinsic personal qualities.

Thus, we feel that it is important that research be undertaken on the nature of the diagnostic process in rehabilitation programs. It seems especially important to document the subsequent effects of labelling on the disability careers of the severely handicapped by following their cases beyond the branching decisions forced upon them by screening outcomes. It would also be of interest to conduct demonstration projects in which the proportion distribution of labels applied is intentionally distorted in favor of marginal clients, whose rehabilitation careers could then be followed to determine, at least indirectly, the social costs of the labelling procedure as it is ordinarily applied. An important related question concerns the patterns that obtain in the application of labels. Do the elderly, the poor, and/or the black and Hispanic clients run higher risks of being classified "incapable of rehabilitation" in programs in which other clients with similar disabilities are not so labelled?

Another research need can only be identified briefly. The reports examined shed little or no light on the important question of the structural and organizational arrangements under which more favorable rehabilitation outcomes occur. Collignon and Serot (1973) conducted an analysis of the impact of "organizational overstructure" on performance of rehabilitation programs. They found that variations in several structural variables had little effect, once certain controls were utilized, upon the efficiency of rehabilitative services or the proportions of successful outcomes thereof. Theirs is an interesting finding, but it is hardly definitive. We suggest that more research be undertaken in regard to organizational arrangements and that replications be considered as a regular part of research policy.

One final comment is in order. We would not wish the reader to believe that the negative findings reported here are peculiar to rehabilitation research focusing on organizational variables. Rather, the poor quality of the research examined here is probably symptomatic of a much broader problem with respect to basic evaluative research on social-action and intervention programs in general. For amplification of these issues, see Martinson, 1974; Bernstein et al., 1973; Mann, 1965.

REFERENCES

Those reports with an asterisk were included in our sample of 477 projects. A complete list of all reports reviewed by the authors is available through the Disability and Health Economics Research Section of the Bureau of Economic Research at Rutgers University.

Argyris, C. "Creating Effective Research Relationships in Organizations." Human Organization 17 (Spring 1958): 34-40.

Aronson, S.H., and Sherwood, C.C. "Researcher Versus Practitioner: Problems in Social Action Research." Social Work 12 (October 1967): 89-96.

Bernstein, I.H., Reiker, P.P., and Freeman, H.E. "A Review of Evaluation Research: The State of the Art, Methodological Practices, and Dissemination of Research Findings." Paper presented at the American Sociological Association Meetings, New York, August 1973.

Campbell, D.T. and Stanley, J.C. Experimental and Quasi-Experimental Designs for Research. Chicago: Rand McNally, 1966.

Collignon, F.C., and Serot, D.E. "An Investigation of the Impact of Organizational Overstructure upon the Performance of State Vocational Rehabilitation Programs." Report submitted to the Vocational Rehabilitation Administration, Department of Social and Health Services, State of Washington, 1973.

*Dibner, A., Nicholas, H., and Goldberg, R.T. The Vocational
    Rehabilitation of Disabled Public Assistance Clients. Boston:
    Massachusetts Rehabilitation Commission.

*Educational Evaluation and Research Associates. The San Antonio
    Rehabilitation-Welfare Final Report on Research and Demon-
    stration. Austin, Tex.: Texas Education Agency, Vocational
    Rehabilitation Division, 1969.

Freeman, H.E. and Sherwood, C.C. "Research in Large-Scale
    Intervention Programs." Journal of Social Issues 21, (January
    1965): 11-21.

Glaser, B.G., and Strauss, A.L. Time for Dying. Chicago: Aldine,
    1968.

Hasenfield, Y., and English, R.A., eds. Human Service Organiza-
    tions. Ann Arbor, Mich.: University of Michigan Press, 1973.

Hovland, C.I. "Reconciling Conflicting Results Derived from Experi-
    mental and Survey Studies of Attitude Change." American
    Psychologist 14 (1959): 8-17.

Mann, J. Changing Human Behavior. New York: Scribner's, 1965.

Martinson, R. "What Works? Questions and Answers About Prison
    Reform." The Public Interest 35 (Spring 1974): 22-52.

*Pagan, A. Vocational Rehabilitation of Disabled Public Welfare
    Clients. Rio Piedras, P.R.: Division of Vocational Rehabilita-
    tion, 1968.

Pelz, D.C. "Some Social Factors Related to Performance in a
    Research Organization." Administrative Science Quarterly 1
    (1956): 310-25.

Rosenhan, D.L. "On Being Sane in Insane Places." Science,
    January 19, 1973, pp. 250-58.

Rosenthal, R., and Jacobson, L. Pygmalion in the Classroom. New
    York: Holt, Reinhart and Winston, 1968.

Roth, J.A. "Some Contingencies of the Moral Evaluation and Control
    of Clientele: The Case of the Hospital Emergency Service."
    American Journal of Sociology 77 (March 1972): 839-56.

*Roth, J.A., and Eddy, E.M. Rehabilitation for the Unwanted. New York: Atherton Press, 1967.

Safilos-Rothschild, C. The Sociology and Social Psychology of Disability and Rehabilitation. New York: Random House, 1970.

Scott, R.A. The Making of Blind Men. New York: Russell Sage Foundation, 1969.

______. "The Selection of Clients by Social Welfare Agencies: The Case of the Blind." Social Problems 14 (Winter 1967): 248-57.

______. Sharples, G.E., and Crawford, R.L. Child Amputees: Disability Outcomes and Antecedents. Ann Arbor, Mich.: University of Michigan, 1972.

Vinter, R.D. "Analysis of Treatment Organizations." Social Work 8 (July 1963): 3-15.

Weiss, C.H. "Methods of Assessing Program Effectiveness." Evaluation Research. Englewood Cliffs, N.J.: Prentice-Hall, 1972.

Wessen, A.F. "The Apparatus of Rehabilitation: An Organizational Analysis." Sociology and Rehabilitation, Marvin B. Sussman, ed. Washington, D.C.: American Sociological Association, 1965.

Williams, W. "The Capacity of Social Science Organization to Perform Large-Scale Evaluation Research." Evaluating Social Programs, Walter Williams and Peter H. Rossi, eds. New York: Seminar Press, 1972.

*Wisconsin Division of Vocational Rehabilitation. Wood County Project. Madison, Wis.: University of Wisconsin.

Zimbardo, P.G. "A Pirandellan Prison." New York Times Magazine, April 8, 1973, pp. 38ff.

13

COST-BENEFIT ANALYSIS IN REHABILITATION AND REHABILITATIONAL RESEARCH

Cost-benefit analysis can be a significant aid in making choices among alternative investment possibilities. In the public sector, much as in the private sector, decision makers need relevant information on which to base their allocation of investment funds. Cost-benefit analysis provides the information necessary to make economically efficient decisions. That form of economic analysis need not be the exclusive component of any decision; a number of other factors can serve both as possible objectives or constraints. In general, though, when all the relevant costs and benefits of an investment are spelled out and compared, the decision maker is in a better position to make the investment choice that will add the most to his objective, while remaining within the bounds formed by his constraints.

COST-BENEFIT ANALYSIS: ITS SCOPE AND LIMITATIONS

In the past decade cost-benefit analysis has been applied to a myriad of social programs. Although the tool has been available for some time, its use had until recently been limited to the evaluation of physical investment. With the development of human capital theory in the 1960s people began to recognize that many social expenditures could reasonably be considered investments. Along with that realization there was an increasing demand for government funds from all sectors of the economy, significantly spurred on by the Vietnam War. That competition for funds was combined with a growing public awareness of social problems and the increasing availability of technical skills to make cost-benefit analysis the logical tool. If, through the use of that method, it could be shown that a program satisfied some pertinent investment criterion, one's demand for funds could be scientifically validated.

How would that validation occur, and why would it be an acceptable argument for the allocation of new or continued funds to a particular endeavor? To answer that, one needs to return to the nature of cost-benefit analysis and what it does. Basically (as one could predict from its name), cost-benefit analysis consists of a comparison between all relevant costs and benefits. Unfortunately, the difficulties we face far outweigh the seemingly simple task of measuring and counting all costs and benefits. The particulars of the problem are discussed later in this chapter. First, we shall attempt to show how cost-benefit analysis can be used to justify expenditures.

Assuming that we can calculate the costs and benefits with certainty, we can then determine the return on a particular investment. Given the decision maker's objective of maximizing the national income, he can attain that end by funding those projects with the greatest potential returns at the margin until all funds are expended.

One flaw in the argument is that its assumptions are unrealistic. In cases where investment returns occur over a period of years there is no way that one can be certain about the magnitude of the returns, especially in the case of human resources. One therefore has to make further calculations based either on past experience or on some other set of incomplete data in order to be able to predict with some certainty the likely outcome of an investment.

The second assumption that needs clarification is that concerning the maximization of national income. That measure is generally acceptable, but a better measure would be the maximization of societal welfare; in cases of human capital investment, a divergence between national income and social welfare results from the impossibility of directly measuring a number of returns.

Another error is the implicit assumption that the only constraint confronting a decision maker is a fiscal constraint. Surely, political and ethical constraints also figure importantly in the decision making process.

Basic to the above discussion of objectives and constraints is the efficiency-equity argument.* The traditional and valid argument of economists is that distributional issues are best ignored in the

---

*It is important to remember that we are dealing here with income distribution. Among the other types of distributions that may be relevant are geography, age, race, and health.

interest of maximizing social welfare; in other words, our decisions should be directed above all toward efficiency. After having attained maximum efficiency, we can make the income transfers necessary to arrive at the income distribution mandated by society.

That construct, although logically correct, may fail to meet the practical exigencies confronting decision makers. For example, an elected official may be wary of the criticism he is certain to receive if he proposes programs that clearly favor the affluent. As a realist, he may be skeptical about the attainment of redistribution according to the economists' plan. Hence, he may choose to base his decision upon some distributional consideration. Unfortunately, since the distributional constraint upon him is seldom explicit, the program's net distributional impact may be a function of many influences other than that of a predetermined distribution.*

An explicit statement of desired distributional consequences is essential, because in many cases equity and efficiency are contradictory objectives. Unless one knows the relationship or the tradeoff possibilities, one cannot adequately determine a funding position. Once funds are allocated, some distributional effect will occur, thereby implicitly indicating our relative preferences for the two goals. It is argued that that judgment should be explicit and prior to funding decisions.

In designing a rehabilitation program for efficiency, our emphasis would be upon reaching those whose net gain from a rehabilitation program would be the greatest. Although literature (see Conley, 1969; Bellante, 1972) is divided on the question of optimal target populations, one can assume that the majority would be comprised of middle-income people. That assumption is based on the observation that the low-income disabled population is typically characterized by low levels of education, little experience, and other attributes that militate against employment success. Since they may have the least to start with, their income stream is unlikely to be improved at all without a major set of expenditures. On the other end of the scale, disabled individuals having a relatively high income stand to gain little from rehabilitation in terms of income.

If our above assumptions are correct, the middle-income class should receive the bulk of rehabilitation expenditures. Assuming that

---

*There are two ways to measure a net distributional effect. One is to gauge the net transfer occurring at a point in time due to a specific program. The other is to measure a program's impact upon distribution over a period of years. While the first is the one most often discussed, it is usually confused with the second, which is the significantly more difficult procedure.

rehabilitation is financed by a proportional tax structure, we would see a net redistribution from the poor and rich to the middle class. If that is society's goal as regards distribution, then we have no problem; if not, however, then we must be willing to sacrifice efficiency or to alter the revenue base to attain the desired distributional impact.

The final decision about any public investment is left to the political process. Cost-benefit analysis supplements the process by making available the information needed for decision making. If that information is incorrectly applied, misused, or ignored, the final choice may differ from that suggested by the cost-benefit analysis; yet that decision may be the best solution for the society as a whole.

Since the decision maker is aware of the need to evaluate a number of noneconomic variables, his final choice will be based on much more information than that provided by a cost-benefit analysis. Such analysis, therefore, needs to be viewed as only one part of a broad range of public decision-making tools and not as the single deciding factor.

Having presented a general description of cost-benefit analysis, we shall now examine some of the specific difficulties involved in a cost-benefit analysis of rehabilitation.

METHODOLOGY AND POLICY UTILITY

We shall begin by considering cost-benefit analysis in terms of some of the questions on the checklist (see the appendix).

Grantee

We note that many cost-benefit studies are not parts of funded projects; in many cases they are conducted after a project or program has been completed. Recently, however, there has been a definite trend toward including the specification of costs and benefits in research projects. One positive outgrowth of that trend is the ability of original researchers to collect more adequate data on costs and benefits.

Two cautionary notes should be sounded here. First, given the special bias of the researcher in determining the costs and benefits of his own program, we shall be leary of accepting any offhand estimates and assumptions. Second, the unique character of every project should alert us to the need for replication and variations in project size. We must reconsider costs and benefits when seemingly similar programs are undertaken with different populations.

Our review of a number of cost-benefit studies leads us to conclude that outside evaluators are needed to assure scientific integrity. Separation between evaluator and researcher is essential if we are to avoid the pitfalls of overlooking some relevant factors or of making assumptions in a cavalier manner in order to corroborate a predetermined goal. It is not altogether clear whether the original grantor of funds should be responsible for selecting the analyst. But it would appear that the commissioning by the original funder of two grants—one for the project and one for the cost-benefit evaluation— would further our goal of independence.

Subject Matter and Handicap

A project's subject matter and the disability of its clients have a pronounced effect upon the calculation of costs and benefits. In almost all cases the rehabilitation process entails some vocational outcome. But for projects whose central objectives improved self-concept or independent lifestyle, a cost-benefit analysis is too monetarily oriented to be of much use. While vocational programs can rely on the job market as a standard for evaluating the skills acquired by a rehabilitated client, no such standard exists for projects whose objectives are nonvocational. Although we can make a partial estimate of homemaker benefits and of the impact of an individual's rehabilitation upon the members of his family, there are far too many nonpecuniary factors at work for us to rely solely upon monetary consideration in our analysis.

Obviously, handicaps vary widely. (Some limitation on what gets done for which people may exist relative to the three possible outcomes discussed above.) In general, many of the more detailed studies cover comprehensive vocational-rehabilitation programs, thereby including a variety of handicaps. (See Collignon and Dodson, 1973; Bellante, 1972; Grigg et al., 1970, as some examples. Cost and benefits are calculated separately for different disability groups.)

One should avoid statements concerning a program's effectiveness in treating all handicaps: What may be a very effective program for one disability group may fail miserably for another. The differences are critical in making future investment decisions. (See Chapter 11 for further discussion.)

Sampling

We must be cautious in the choice of a study group. Were we to select only those most likely to achieve rehabilitation, we would face innumerable difficulties in trying to generalize results for similar programs with more varied populations. (One example of that kind of problem is in Wright and Reagles [1971]. The study is in a county that is mainly rural and white. Trying to make generalizations of program success for the disadvantaged in other areas with different economies and clients is very dangerous.) Generalizability also depends on the "sameness" of programs. Clearly, a program's specific benefit-cost ratio cannot be applied to another program unless the latter is essentially the same as the former. Although we can compare ratios over distinct programs for decision purposes, we cannot assume that one ratio will hold for different programs.

Follow-Up

Follow-up is an important factor in determining benefits. To calculate benefits, it is essential that we know the length of a client's job tenure. And since the salary associated with a job is the major benefit of rehabilitation, we also need earnings data over time both for rehabilitants and for a similar group of people, categorized by significant characteristics, who did not receive services. That comparison is necessary for a true measure of the change produced by rehabilitation, for only through such comparative evaluation can we gain a clear notion of how successful a client would have been had he not received services.

The control of demographic, rehabilitation-related, and socio-economic variables is of major concern to a cost-benefit analyst. The impact of those variables upon earnings must be recognized so that we can separate out the true effects of rehabilitation. For example, age, sex, education, occupational experience and skills, and severity of disability can all alter the earning power of an individual. One attempt to hold some of these factors constant is found in Bellante (1972). Through the use of regression analysis he measures the impact of ten variables, not only on success but also on productivity and cost.*

---

*His ten variables are age, sex, race, education, major type of disability, presence of a secondary disability, public-assistance status, type of residence, marital status, and number of dependents. A similar type of analysis is found in Grigg et al. (1970).

Another statistical tool used increasingly often in cost-benefit studies is sensitivity analysis. That method, which we shall later discuss in greater detail, enables us to see the effect our assumptions can have on our conclusions.

COST-BENEFIT ANALYSIS AND REHABILITATION

We shall now explore some specific difficulties associated with performing cost-benefit analysis in the rehabilitation field. We have isolated six major problem areas: perspective; pre- and postproject earnings; choice of a discount rate; adjustments for postproject labor-force changes; use of a ratio; and measurement of costs.

Perspective

Relevant benefits and costs depend on the one on whose behalf the study is being conducted. Since the results are to be used in making some investment decision, the data correspond to those costs and benefits relevant to the decision-making unit. Society is the unit to be considered if some overall change in welfare is sought. Other possible decision-making units are local, state, or federal governments; a public agency; the individual or his family; and the employer of the rehabilitant.

For society, the analysis takes into account all real resource costs and all benefits, both to individuals and to society as a whole; that is the broadest perspective one can take. It should take into account all the external effects (externalities) resulting from the public investment under study.* In practice, however, we are prevented from attaining all the desired information by the nonexistence of markets. That means that market prices cannot be used to measure the value or benefit of the goods for each consumer. That market failure (public goods, externalities, and imperfect capital markets) is the major economic justification for government intervention in the rehabilitation field.

---

*Externalities are defined as costs or benefits that do not accrue to the specific unit; they are generally not considered by the individual consuming or producing unit when making an investment or consumption decision.

If the decision-making perspective shifts from that of society as a whole to that of the agency or the individual, it will be easier to measure costs and benefits. For example, for an individual the total costs are simply how much he pays for services combined with the indirect or opportunity costs involved in his taking time off to participate. His true measure of benefit would be obtained from knowing the market price and his demand curve for rehabilitation, but we are forced to substitute as a proxy the change in his lifetime earnings due to rehabilitation.* The reader is urged to consider the many other cases where the factors entering into the calculation of costs and benefits differ, depending upon the nature of the decision maker.

Pre- and Postproject Earnings

The most common measure of benefits is the change in an individual's earnings resulting from his rehabilitation. Unfortunately, the true change is not readily identifiable; without either a well-matched control group or prior data we are unable to attribute earnings to specific factors, such as rehabilitation. Economists are now attempting to measure the effects upon earnings of schooling, experience, and other variables (Mincer, 1974). Their measurements are made possible by the availability of both sophisticated statistical techniques and abundant data on individual situations over a long period of time. Such data do not exist in the case of rehabilitated/not-rehabilitated disabled persons.

A major difficulty in estimating the net change in earnings attributable to rehabilitation is the determination of prerehabilitation earnings. That determination is obviously necessary if we are to derive some measure of rehabilitation impact. Earnings at entry are biased because people usually seek the services of a rehabilitation agency when they are doing poorly. Certainly, there is no "correct" time span for obtaining measure of prerehabilitation earnings. A

---

*Since an individual's demand curve illustrates the value he places on a certain quantity of goods, the schedule would give us a measure of how much an individual personally values a certain amount of rehabilitation. Given imperfections and lack of private markets, we are forced to try to determine an individual's demand curve from available information; earnings due to rehabilitation is the factor that we generally choose.

weekly earnings average over the previous year might provide an
adequate and representative measure; we could use those earnings
as a basis for projecting future earnings had the client not been rehabilitated. We have no way of knowing exactly how much a client would
have improved his productivity on his own. Only by analyzing data
on a random control group, classified according to a number of
personal and vocational characteristics, and covering a substantial
period of years, could we hope to predict outcomes in the absence of
rehabilitation.

On the postrehabilitation side we face similar problems in
establishing the optimum length of time after rehabilitation on which
to base conclusions about a change in earnings. Again, data over a
long period of time for a number of rehabilitants classified by a
variety of characteristics—e.g., time in rehabilitation, services
received, severity of disability, attitude, education, age, sex, and
prior skills—could be very useful in predicting individual benefits
from rehabilitation. Given that information, we could judge the effectiveness of rehabilitation in terms of improved earnings. We must
gauge the earnings change attributable to rehabilitation, if we are to
measure benefits and make recommendations for efficient funding.*

Choice of a Discount Rate

In choosing a discount rate it is most critical that we recognize
why the choice is necessary. For a number of reasons (uncertainty,
inflation, and a time-rate of preference) a dollar today is worth more
than one dollar in the future. To account for the divergence we must
"devalue" or discount future dollars to the present. The choice of a
discount rate is important in that it may very well alter the balance
of investment between the public and private sectors.

According to the concept of opportunity costs: "It follows almost
immediately that the correct discount rate for the evaluation of a
government project is the percentage rate of return that the resources
utilized would otherwise provide in the private sector" (emphasis in

---

*One factor we have not explicitly considered but that deserves
mention is employer contributions to social security and other
employee-related programs. Those are certainly benefits to the
employee, and their existence makes earnings an imperfect measure
of the return from rehabilitation.

original) (Baumol, 1970, p. 274). Long-term government or corporate bonds offer some possible measures of the rate of return. Although they do not provide a true measure of opportunity cost (we would need to know the exact source of government revenue), they certainly are more satisfactory than a rate chosen only because others have used it. If one seeks comparisons between the project at hand and an earlier project, it is best that one use the most appropriate rate for both, rather than the rate used in the earlier report.

Uncertainty about the best rate to use can be resolved through sensitivity analysis (see Berkowitz and Anderson, 1974, p. 113; Collignon and Dodson, 1973, p. 49). By varying the discount rate along with the rest of the given data, we can discover how the magnitude of the rate affects our conclusions. Sensitivity analysis also enables us to see the discount rate necessary to assure project efficiency. The rate would be of interest if one were concerned with providing for future generations (a low discount rate would mean a preference for longer projects). By seeing how low a rate we need, we give society a measure of the cost of providing for future generations.

Labor Force-Participation Adjustments

One reason we cannot use earnings at closure as a measure of rehabilitation benefit extended over an individual's remaining work life is that that figure does not encompass a number of factors that detract from his full employment over the period. For example, the death of an individual between closure and retirement would certainly decrease the expected benefit from rehabilitation. Although the probabilities for such occurrences are estimated in standard life tables, the special characteristics of the disabled make it difficult to choose the appropriate probability.

In addition, a recurrence of the disability might also offset employment benefits. The size of this factor depends heavily upon both the nature of the previous disability and the type of job in which the client is employed.

Another labor-force adjustment that needs consideration is the possibility of unemployment during the period from closure to retirement. Although we do not know whether or not the rehabilitated have a greater unemployment probability than the rest of the population, we would do well to account for the possibility of periods of unemployment. Our concern, as always, in measuring that factor should be with the differential between the duration of unemployment without rehabilitation and that with rehabilitation. We can thereby derive

some measure of the net effect of rehabilitation on unemployment
and upon eventual earnings.

Employer attitudes may also require an adjustment. Are the
rehabilited discriminated against in a manner similar to the poor,
the nonwhite, the low skilled? Are they the last hired and the first
fired? The question of possible job discrimination deserves further
economic analysis, not merely another study of employers' attitudes.*

Another labor-related adjustment concerns changes in an individual's productivity. We assume that an individual's capacity (and,
thus, his earning power) increases as he learns on the job and as his
working conditions improve. Since we have earnings data for only a
short period following rehabilitation, we must adjust future earnings
to allow for productivity changes. And similar adjustments must be
made in calculating the estimated earnings of the nonrehabilitated.
Whether the potential productivity changes in those two cases are the
same may depend on the type of rehabilitation services performed
and the nature of the work the person is doing or would have done.
(Our guess is that the rehabilitant's productivity increases with the
rest of the economy, while the nonrehabilitant has a lower productivity
potential.)

Problems in Using a Benefit-Cost Ratio

The traditional criterion for efficient investment in rehabilitation has been the benefit-cost ratio. One of the problems posed by
its use concerns the size of the projects available. Suppose we find
that the benefit-cost ratios for a set of projects $X_1 \ldots X_n$ are all
> 1 with the ratio for $X_1 > X_2$ and so on, with $X_2 > X_3 \ldots > X_n$.
That does not necessarily mean that we should invest our money in
X_1, although, taken by itself, it would give us the greatest return
per dollar; the fact that we are operating under a budget constraint
would necessitate our ruling out project X_1 at the scale considered,
if its cost exceeded our available funds. If we reduced the size of
X_1 in order to satisfy our constraint, we cannot be certain that the

---

*One way in which discrimination against the disabled can
manifest itself has a parallel in our national pasttime. Baseball
owners argue that they do not hire a black manager because of the
adverse criticism that would result should it become necessary to
fire him. Possible employers of the handicapped could use a similar
line of reasoning in justifying their refusal to hire the disabled.

ratio for X_1 will still be greater than that for X_2. In other words, we do not know the precise effects of a project's scale upon its ratio.

A theoretical solution would be to invest our money in all available projects, shifting funds among projects until the last dollar spent on each project yields the same marginal or extra benefits, thus maximizing our overall return. Unfortunately, such a procedure is completely impracticable, since the indivisibility of research projects precludes the shifting of funds. If we were able to "buy" small units of several research projects, we could not be certain about their respective benefit-cost ratios. The only alternative, then, would be to invest in available projects, each of a restricted size.

Measurement of Costs

Two major difficulties arise with respect to measuring costs. The first involves deciding the costs that are relevant. (That will, of course, depend on the study's perspective.) The second concerns the mechanics of measuring the costs. From the perspective of society, for example, all real resource costs are important. In other words, any component of a program that is taken from its prior use entails a cost to society. We measure that cost in terms of its alternative uses—i.e., its opportunity cost.

We shall now examine some relevant examples of the cost aspects of a rehabilitation program as viewed from society's perspective. If we assume that the disabled individual spends a full day at a rehabilitation center, we assume that he can no longer be engaged in productive work, and hence he and society incur a cost. Another example is that of transfer payments. The decline in transfers to welfare recipients and the unemployed is not a real gain to society, since it merely involves a resource <u>transfer</u>. But from the individual's perspective, a loss of welfare payments represent a cost and must be accounted for as such in his investment decision. All direct and many indirect services provided during rehabilitation represent a resource used—i.e., a cost. Furthermore, where the services of more than one agency are involved, their costs must be included in the overall calculation.

One cost that is often included but about which we have reservations is that relating to research and demonstrations. There is undoubtedly a cost required to operate the programs, but the question is whether some percentage of the cost should be included in a cost-benefit analysis of a national vocational-rehabilitation program. If we include part of the costs, how can we justify not "paying" for all the knowledge we so used? In other words, once a project is completed, the information it contains becomes a "public good" and can be used equally by anyone at no cost other than that required to obtain the information.

When many people use the results stemming from a project, the possibility of double counting exists. For example, suppose ten VR programs used one-tenth of the knowledge, and, hence, incurred one-tenth of the cost, of a research program. Why should the eleventh agency be treated differently? And yet if we do not treat it differently, we shall be "overpaying" and underinvesting. We maintain that the decision whether or not to invest in a rehabilitation program should not even be related to the use made of research results. Since the research costs are in essence sunk costs, they should have no bearing on our decision. We are thus arguing that separate decisions be made regarding the investment feasibility of rehabilitation and rehabilitation research with the costs of the latter not included in the benefit-cost analysis of the former. (Conley [1969, p. 241] on the other hand, defends the inclusion of those research costs when one is working in a broad societal scope.)

The costs of research and demonstration projects do become relevant in the decision of whether or not to undertake the research. In estimating the possible benefits of the research, we may include not only the immediate benefits discovered during the project but also the potential benefits anticipated from the knowledge produced. One problem we face here is in trying to determine whether the knowledge would have been available without the project.

BENEFIT-COST RESULTS AND THEIR USES

Benefit-cost ratios vary widely, depending upon the perspective, the methodology, and the clientele under consideration. Ratios can vary from 70:1 (Wood County, 1971) to 18:1 (Michigan, 1971) to much lower or even negative results. Given ratios that indicate a substantial investment return, how can we implement the data for the most efficient allocation of funds?

Since results differ from one client group to another, it is essential to calculate ratios for alternative populations. A state agency, whose only constraint was a limited budget could afford to invest (i.e., provide rehabilitation services similar to those analyzed in the benefit-cost analysis) in the group offering the highest return. But the scale of operation remains a relevant factor. If a project, after serving X clients, experiences a decline in population that eliminates everyone but the "hard-core," we can expect benefit-cost rankings to alter. A reexamination of its position would show that the greatest return might be from a different group and type of service. If the financial constraint is relatively weak, the agency will wind up serving a variety of groups with different programs but with relatively similar benefit-cost ratios.

The "real-world" problem is that we cannot make pariahs out of a group because it generates a low benefit-cost ratio, even though, in terms of the national economy, it might be more efficient to do so. Since, practically speaking, we must invest in all groups, it is imperative for us to be fully aware of the effectiveness of different programs for people with similar handicaps. Such awareness will allow greater leeway in obtaining the best return on our investment while still meeting the needs of a broad spectrum of the disabled.

ECONOMIC ANALYSIS OF REHABILITATION RESEARCH

This section raises two important questions. First how can we most efficiently allocate research funds, given a set of proposed projects? Second, how valuable, in terms of costs and benefits, has a given research project been? Those two questions are obviously related. Better understanding of the first can make for better projects in the second. Knowledge of the hows and whys of economically successful projects can help us in the future allocation of funds. Up to now little consideration has been given to those questions. Research in the area has been either preliminary (Thrall, 1973) or theoretical (Nerlove, 1972), and it has had limited practicability for rehabilitation (Grossfield and Heath, 1966; Griliches, 1958).

In the preproject stage our objective is to obtain the best possible notion of the potential costs and returns from a diverse set of projects. Since the projects are in the proposal stage, we can more easily secure information about their costs than we can about their chances of success and the implications of their results. The Analytic Aids for Research Proposal Selection (AARPS) report discusses ordinal and cardinal measurements. (The final choice of programs, given their rank and existing fiscal constraints, would be similar to the stepwise process described in our discussion of cost-benefit analysis).

An ordinal ranking tells us whether one project is preferred to another, but since it does not assign values to the projects, it does not tell us the degree to which one is preferable to another. The ranking does, however, provide us with some measure by which to allocate funds.

A revised ordinal model is as follows:

$$S = P_s \, (V_b + V_i \, P_u)$$

where S is project score; P_s is the probability of success; V_b is the benefits expected from a successful project; V_i is the degree to which the project aids in the resolution of a specified issue; P_u is the probability of the results being utilized (Allen et al., 1973). The problem with that type of model is that it requires subjective judgments based on imperfect knowledge. But, through the use of a Delphi method, previously recognized aspects of good research, and the involvement of knowledgeable SRS staff, we can have informed input in the decisions responsible for determining the rankings. Fortunately or unfortunately (depending upon one's view), the model has the capacity to incorporate the political constraints so important to decision making. Another drawback of the model—one that militates against relying exclusively on its ranking—is its lack of concern for the magnitude of costs and benefits. The decision maker may be left in a quandary as to whether or not the highest-ranking project will actually produce the most efficient allocation of research funds.

The cardinal model, as developed at the Texas Institute, attempts a numerical calculation of the possible benefits associated with a research project—clearly, a more difficult task. The proposed model is as follows:

$$B = P_s \, (P_u NB_i + B_s) + B_f$$

where B is the expected benefits; P_s is the same as above; P_u is the probability of utilization; N is the number of people in the target group; B_i is the per-individual benefit of a successful project; B_s is the indirect benefits; B_f is the benefit of funding the research, even if unsuccessful (Thrall 1973). Although the model also requires subjective evaluations, they can be minimized by prior knowledge of results of completed projects, thereby allowing for statistical predictions.

One consideration missing from the model is the time span over which benefits accrue. The model can be specified without a time span, but, certainly, no calculations of a project's ultimate benefits and costs of a project can be made without that relevant information. We need such information in order to establish whether and when the possible results of the research would have otherwise become available to practitioners. Projects whose results derive from traditional procedures will have a relatively short time span over which benefits accrue, whereas those whose results accrue from innovative methods may not realize over a long period of time.

Again, the allocation of funds based on the model may result in the adoption of only a few expensive projects. If no political constraint limits the number of projects to be funded, the most efficient solution would be to allocate funds based on the ratios, until the fiscal constraint is met.*

Further development, specification, and testing of the models are needed. The testing of how well the models rank projects is necessarily a postproject task.† We need a standard procedure for seeing how well we can predict a project's success and its potential benefits. We could then compare our predictions for all projects in a given year (ex post results) with the rankings derived from the two models. It is doubtful that the correlation would be high; some modification would certainly be necessary in order to formulate a model with reasonably accurate predictive capacity.

CONCLUSIONS

Several problems face the evaluator attempting to undertake a cost-benefit analysis of a rehabilitation program or research project. Although we have not been overly specific about cost-benefit studies (a number of them are listed in the reference section), we have attempted to draw from the studies examples of the most critical problems. The reader should now understand that cost-benefit analysis is an intricate tool subject to numerous data problems and vagaries resulting from the requisite assumptions. Since its sole concern is economic efficiency (assuming the inability to incorporate an equity constraint) cost-benefit analysis cannot be used alone in the decision

---

*There is less of a scale problem relative to rehabilitation research than there is relative to rehabilitation, since research may well be an all-or-nothing activity.

†Two attempts to do ex post analysis of the cost and benefits of research in agriculture are found in Griliches (1958) and in Grossfield and Heath (1966). The former attempts to measure the social rate of return on expenditures for hybrid-corn research. The technique is to divide "the estimated perpetual flow of returns . . . by the cumulated research expenditures to arrive at a rate of return that will equalize the present value of the flow of returns with the cumulated value of research expenditures" (Griliches, 1958, p. 419). He estimates that as of 1955 there was at least a 700-percent annual return on each dollar invested in hybrid-corn research.

making process. Also involved in the investment decision are a number of other factors whose net import offset any reductions in economic efficiency that they might well entail.

Attempts to measure the benefits and costs of research deserve further study. Presently, little is known about the future payoffs and likely successes of research projects. Refinement of the efficiency approach to funding research will result in improved allocation by reducing the impact of subjective factors.

REFERENCES

Allen, J.R., Fuhrer, M.J., Spencer, W.A., and Moffet, C.L. Proposed Procedures for Prioritizing the F.Y.-74 SRS Research Project Proposals and Guidelines. Analytic Aids for Research Proposal Selection. Report no. 73-9. Houston, Tex.: Texas Institute for Rehabilitation and Research, 1973.

Averous, C., Stahl, K., and Cole, C. Cost-Benefit Analysis of Rehabilitation Services Programs: A First Model and its Sensitivity Analysis. Berkeley, Calif.: University of California, Berkeley, 1971.

Baumol, W.J. "On the Discount Rate for Public Projects." In Public Expenditures and Policy Analysis, Robert Haveman and Julius Margolis, eds. Chicago: Markham, 1970.

Bellante, D.M. "A Multivariate Analysis of a Vocational Rehabilitation Program." Journal of Human Resources 7 (1972): 226-41.

Berkowitz, M., and Anderson, M. PADEC—An Evaluation of an Experimental Rehabilitation Project. New Brunswick, N.J.: Disability and Health Economics Research Section, Bureau of Economic Research, Rutgers University, 1974.

Burkhead, J., and Miner, J. Public Expenditure. Chicago: Aldine, 1971.

Campbell, D., and Stanley, J. Experimental and Quasi-Experimental Designs for Research. Chicago: Rand McNally 1963.

Collignon, F.C. A Working Outline for Cost-Benefit Analysis of Vocational Rehabilitation Programs. Berkeley, Calif.: Institute of Urban and Regional Development, University of California, Berkeley, 1971.

______. and Dodson, R. Cost-Benefit Analysis of the Vocational Rehabilitation Programs of the State of Washington. Berkeley, Calif.: Berkeley Planning Associates, 1973.

Conley, R.W. "Benefit-Cost Analysis and Vocational Rehabilitation." In Research Utilization in Rehabilitation Facilities, Ralph Pacinelli, ed. Washington, D.C.: The International Association of Rehabilitation Facilities, 1971.

______. "A Benefit-Cost Analysis of the Vocational Rehabilitation Programs." Journal of Human Resources 4 (1969): 226-52.

Conley, R. The Economics of Mental Retardation. Baltimore, Md.: Johns Hopkins University Press, 1973.

______. The Economics of Vocational Rehabilitation. Baltimore, Md.: Johns Hopkins University Press, 1965.

Grigg, C., Holtman, A., and Martin, P. Vocational Rehabilitation for the Disadvantaged: An Economic and Sociological Evaluation. Lexington, Mass.: Heath, 1970.

Griliches, Z. "Research Costs and Social Returns: Hybrid Corn and Related Innovations." Journal of Political Economy 66 (October 1958): 419-31.

Grossfield, K., and Heath, J.B. "The Benefit and Cost of Government Support for Research and Development: A Case Study." Economic Journal 76 (September 1966): 537-49.

Marglin, S.A. Public Investment Criteria: Benefit-Cost Analysis for Planned Economic Growth. Cambridge, Mass.: MIT Press, 1967.

Mars, L.I., U.S. Department of Health, Education, and Welfare, Statistics and Studies. An Exploratory Cost-Benefit Analysis of Vocational Rehabilitation. Washington, D.C.: Government Printing Office, 1967.

Millward, R. Public Expenditure Economics—An Introductory Application of Welfare Economics. London: McGraw-Hill, 1971.

Mincer, J. Schooling, Experience and Earnings. New York: Columbia University Press, 1974.

Musgrave, R.A., and Musgrave, P.B. Public Finance in Theory and
     Practice. New York: McGraw-Hill, 1973.

Nerlove, M. "On Tuition and the Costs of Higher Education: Pro-
     legomena to a Conceptual Framework." Journal of Political
     Economy 80 (May-June 1972): S178-S218.

Struthers, R.D. The Vocational Status of Michigan Rehabilitants of
     Fiscal Year 1969—Two Years After Case Closure. Michigan
     Department of Education, Division of Vocational Rehabilitation,
     1971.

Thrall, R.M. Which Proposed Research Should SRS Support—An
     Application for Benefit/Cost Analysis. Houston, Tex.: Texas
     Institute for Rehabilitation and Research, 1973.

Wright, G., and Reagles, D. The Economic Impact of an Expanded
     Program of Vocational Rehabilitation. Wisconsin Studies in
     Vocational Rehabilitation, monograph 15, series 2. Madison,
     Wis.: University of Wisconsin, 1971.

The purpose of this chapter is threefold: First, we shall
examine in a theoretical way some of the factors that may affect
the quality of research; second, we shall review some proposed
measures of quality; finally, we shall analyze our data to see whether
any relationships exist between quality and a variety of hypothesized
independent variables.

DIFFICULTIES OF EXPERIMENTAL RESEARCH
IN REHABILITATION

The research and demonstration projects in rehabilitation are
designed to test whether a particular method, treatment, or instrument is more effective than another. That is not an easy task, since
it is usually difficult to discern what would have occurred in the
absence of the innovation.

One method to eliminate the uncertainty about the effectiveness
of an innovation is to adopt an experimental design in which everything
is held constant except the new treatment, instrument or method.
By doing that, it becomes possible to identify a cause-and-effect
relationship. Unfortunately, however, the necessary control is not
always available or consistent with existing constraints. For example,
in many cases administrators of programs are reluctant to "stick to
the rules" of experimental design. Many program directors do not
like to be told how to run their projects. If their objective is not one
of purely scientific research, many other factors will enter their
decisions on program design, likely to result in less than perfect
experimental procedure. And the frequent tendency of administrators

to change parts of the program as it progresses also weakens any conclusions one could draw about the true effectiveness of the treatment.

Furthermore, in projects involving people, many things cannot be held constant as is required when adhering to many experimental designs. A number of factors that act on people are outside the range of most project designs. One possible solution to this problem lies in the use of control groups. The use of control groups in social experiments is subject to severe criticism. Opponents cite that their use usually implies depriving the control groups of the treatment. Another reason for the avoidance of control groups is that political expediency frequently dictates that programs be designed on the basis of need, merit; and first-come, first-served, rather than on considerations of experimental adequacy (Rivlin, 1971).

Those arguments do not stand up to rational scrutiny. For instance, a control group need not be deprived of treatment for all time. At the conclusion of the program, if the treatment has been shown successful, there is no reason for the continued denial of services to the control group. Moreover, given the condition that the experiment usually involves an unproven treatment and, hence, may eventually be shown to be ineffective, it is possible that the control group, having received no treatment, may wind up better off. And there is the possibility that rather than comparing a new program with nothing, one can compare it to existing programs; in such cases, the control group is not deprived of services or treatment.

Another, more useful, criticism can be found in the work of Peter Rossi (Rossi and Williams, 1972), who suggests that, in many cases, the random assignment of people to experimental and control groups is misleading. Although randomization theoretically eliminates self-selection biases, in practice, programs are not likely to be free of those biases. According to Rossi, some projects should be evaluated on the basis of the combined effects of self-selection and the program. The result would be an evaluation of programs as they exist in the real world. In other words, since various selection biases occur, it is less misleading to include them in our experiment than to attempt to eliminate them through the randomization process.

The project participants themselves can be the source of difficulties regarding the generalizability of the program. For example, both clients and rehabilitation workers may behave differently in a small-scale experiment than they would in a large-scale or national program. And there is the further possibility of the existence of a Hawthorne effect.

The fact that many social experiments do not have clearly specified goals presents problems for evaluators of such programs, who are then forced to infer measurable goals from general statements about the program. Should the result be a negative evaluation, administrators and policy makers can always argue that the program is effective in terms of "other" goals. Also, the fact that goals are not specified hinders the achievement of quality research. The object is to find the best method for attaining certain goals; without goals, the methods have no direction. Despite the achievement of favorable outcome, the research methodology is not of top quality.

PROPOSED MEASURES OF QUALITY

We shall now review three major attempts to measure the methodological quality of research. Their tools and measures will be compared with those we have developed for our analysis of rehabilitation research. The two studies to be considered at length are Methodological Adequacy of Federal R&D Projects by Willy DeGeyndt (hereafter referred to as WDG) and A Review of Evaluation Research: The State of the Art, Methodological Practices, and Dissemination of Research Findings by Bernstein, Rieker, and Freeman (hereafter referred to as BRF).

WDG developed an instrument to be used by raters who were specially chosen for the review process. The questionnaire, which dealt mainly with methodological issues, raised specific questions about design, sample, statistics, reporting, and overall quality. Attempts were made to acknowledge and account for the biases of various raters (see WDG rater-bias report).

BRF used a somewhat different approach to the measurement of quality. (No approach can be too different, since only a limited number of variables significantly affect methodological quality). They constructed an index based on the quality of methodological procedures used to measure process or input. Among the measurement-related variables covered in their statistical review were the sampling procedures, the type of statistical analysis, and the nature of the data. Some attempt was made to weight the index in cases where there was more sophisticated statistical analysis.*

---

*The index used involved giving a numerical score of 0 to X for a number of categories, with X being equal to the number of items in a group. The less sophisticated techniques were scored at the low end. The score was then weighted by $1/m - 1$, where m was the number of "response categories" (m = X + 1 from the prior sentence). The total scores for their various indexes was "the sum

For our report, reviewers or panel members judged reports on the basis of the checklist summaries and, in most cases, the actual report. As discussed in Chapter 1, the checklist dealt with methodology, data analysis, external validity, and policy utility. By using a dual rating system, we tried to avoid the difficulties involved in attempts to separate the effects of policy and methodology on an overall quality rating. That enabled us to separate the methodological quality of a project from its possible usefulness to practitioners. The importance of the schema is confirmed in the review of Muthard's work below.

In both the WDG and BRF cases the meaning of quality is basically a methodological one; each evidences great concern with design and analysis. Theoretically, projects that failed to meet generally accepted scientific norms would rate lower than those with better design and analysis, but even the best design schemes were subject to the havoc wrought by problems of rater bias, missing information, and special situational difficulties. No doubt the infancy of research in the field is responsible for our inability to handle all the questions satisfactorily.

A second qualitative standard was that of the so-called impact of a piece of research. In BRF's impact index, which accounts for the degree to which a program achieves its specified goals, the variables included are research design, measurement techniques applied, and the generalizability of results as indicated by the representativeness of the sample. BRF went on to combine impact (output) with process (input) variables to obtain an overall measure of quality. They also continued to use the weighting scheme discussed earlier.

A more literal construction of impact can be found in the work of Muthard and associates (Muthard et al., 1973), who attempted to measure impact in terms of four variables: spread, spillover, continuity, and spinoff. To be exact in the meaning of those terms we quote directly (p. 18):

> Spread—the extent to which a project was adopted or
> replicated in other settings;
> Spillover—a project's effectiveness in attracting
> attention and action to peripheral problems related to
> the central focus of the original project;
> Continuity—the extent to which a research program or
> service program received continued financial support

---

of the products of the response code times the weight for each term"
(BRF, Appendix D).

from a local, state, Federal or private agency after the
original funding was exhausted;
Spinoff—the adoption or adaption of procedures, methods,
instruments, or equipment developed for the original
project for any other purposes, especially their use by
other programs or practitioners.

Given the present stage of the development of impact measurement, it is impossible to identify the precise effects of a project.
Rather than try to design a numerical scale, the Muthard study
assigned a field consultant to each of the projects for a summariza-
tion based on survey responses and discussions with project staff
and users of the study. Hence, impact was not rated but rather described and documented, with examples of adoptions of practices,
new legislation, and so on. A significant conclusion of the Muthard
study was that methodological shortcomings did not tend to impede
project impact.

The foregoing has highlighted the conflicts and confusions that
arise when one tries to measure the quality of research. The researcher's definition of quality will depend upon the many and varied
objectives of the projects under study as well as upon the reviewer's
efforts to solve a certain problem or answer a specific question. The
distinction between WDG's and Muthard's notions of quality points up
this controversy: Who is to say that the methodological adequacy of
a report rates above or below its impact? The decision is necessarily
based on the individual's background and perspective. By separating
policy utility from methodology, we hope to provide the reader with
a choice between alternative measures of quality.

FACTORS HYPOTHESIZED AS
AFFECTING QUALITY

Before analyzing our data we shall attempt to specify the
potential effect of certain variables upon the measurement of quality.
The determination of statistical relationships between some of the
independent variables and quality rating would have a number of uses.
For example, foreknowledge of the factors that affect quality can help
grantors allocate funds more effectively. And research grantees can
incorporate into their project design those variables that have been
shown to improve research quality. Finally, such information can
help assure that projects are undertaken by the right people, with
proper methods to achieve high-quality research.

Grantor

The funding agency is likely to have some impact on the quality
of research. Different grantors have different requirements as to
procedures, reporting, and proposal review. For example, strict
proposal review and monitoring may eliminate poor projects, thus
resulting in a positive relationship between grantor and quality. Other
agencies that are less strict and/or operate in an area or discipline
where research is in early stages might exert a negative influence
upon quality.

Two difficulties present themselves in terms of quality and
grantor. First, alternative definitions of quality may imply different
relationships between grantor and quality. If the definition of quality
were based more upon impact than upon methodological adequacy, a
number of different funding aspects would come into play. Second,
the value of finding the existence of a relationship between grantor and
quality may be limited from a policy standpoint. That limitation is
especially severe when we assume that the allocation of funds to
grantor agencies is a given. (BRF did not include grantor as a
variable in their study, not because grantor was found to be insignificant, but because it is not an easily manipulated variable.)

Grantee

The type of organization undertaking the research affects
quality in a number of ways, among them, the type of personnel
employed and the incentives provided. BRF found that universities
generated the "best" research in their sample, whereas profit-making
corporations tended to produce research of lower quality. Here again,
the working definition of quality used is important. For example, if
the standard is methodological adequacy, universities and associated
medical institutions would rate high, since there is strong peer control through promotions and journal publications. But if the emphasis
is upon impact, then the highest rating would go to agencies that
serve people and help practitioners develop their expertise.

Duration and Funding

A project's time span may affect its eventual quality as follows:
Too short a time period could produce inconclusive findings resulting

from a lack of preparation, experimentation, and follow-up; too long a span could generate undue complications stemming from an overload of input that makes it difficult to interpret relationships between input and output variables. In the economists' jargon, we face increasing returns to time at early stages and decreasing returns at later stages.

BRF found that high-quality research most often occurred in studies that were funded for three or more years—a finding that is somewhat contradictory to our theory of decreasing returns. One possible explanation is that the studies of longer duration generally carried higher stipends, thereby indicating a correlation between funding and duration. That funding factor might interfere with the duration effect.

Neither BRF nor WDG found any significant relationship between quality and the amount of project funding. WDG suggested that both funding and duration operate on quality indirectly, by means of intervening variables. We will attempt to separate the effects of those variables in a regression analysis presented later in this chapter.

Discipline

The discipline in which a study is conducted can affect the quality of research. BRF concluded that psychology tended to generate higher quality studies than the other academic disciplines because psychologists are more strongly oriented toward experimentation. Another explanation for differential quality among disciplines is that they possess varying methodological skills because of their experience with funded projects in the past. Moreover, certain areas may simply be more suitable to design techniques.

Other Variables

A variable that may be of significance (but one we did not pursue) is the project's funding: whether as a grant or as a contract.* For example, BRF found that higher quality was associated with grants than with contracts; the variable was a strong predictor of quality

---

*The basic difference between a grant and a contract is the initiating party. Grants are requested by researchers to investigate problems of their own choosing, while contracts are offered by the government for particular research projects.

in the BRF case. One possible explanation of that finding is that scientists are more highly motivated when they work on studies of their own choosing.

Unfortunately, BRF's results were not confirmed in the sample reviewed by WDG. In that case, although the sample was inadequate for statistical inferences (there being only a small number of contracts), a trend was discernible, indicating slightly higher technical quality for contracts than grants.

In our study, two of the additional variables that could be used to explain our panel members' ratings were disability of the clients in the sample under study and subject matter.* One possibility we considered was that the policy utility of a piece of research could be affected by the size of the population at risk relative to the research. A second likelihood was that better-quality research may be taking place in certain disability categories due to their more highly developed research techniques.

Other variables on our checklist that might have influenced our quality ratings (see Chapter 1 and Appendix A) are sampling procedures, statistical analysis, and experimental design. Our sample of research projects will be examined to see how closely they meet the methodological standards established for generalizing and replicating their results.

On the other hand, experimental design may influence the quality of a study in the policy-utility sense. For instance, if a report does not employ a design or use appropriate statistical procedures, its results may not be generalizable. That, in turn, would diminish its usefulness for practitioners.

DATA-BASE LIMITATIONS

Since the sources of our data have been described earlier, we need only reiterate a few points here. Our panel members who were responsible for the methodology and policy-utility ratings were from Rutgers University or nearby colleges and universities. The biases created by having each report rated only once by a panel member from the relevant discipline were discussed and analyzed in Chapter 1. Some other limitations to our data base deserve mention. First, our measures of quality may not adequately account for the quality of

---

*Subject matter refers to the particular rehabilitation process under study; it generally includes intake, type of services, and outcome variables.

demonstration projects; such projects are not necessarily designed to adhere to good scientific methodology. Whether demonstrations should thus be exempt from the strictest of methodological rules depends upon their objectives. WDG suggests that the exemption decision be based upon the category under which the demonstration project falls: a) experimental projects designed to test relationships between variables, b) developmental projects designed to install a proven program in an operating system, or c) feasibility demonstrations designed to test a program in a generalized operational environment. Since the first and third types contain research components to the extent that they adhere to methodological rules, they should be subjected to evaluation.

Another shortcoming of our data results from the screening criteria that were used to limit our sample size. The screening was mainly on the basis of topic, leaving us with a sample representative of only a portion of rehabilitation research. Also, although we did not exclude reports, because we felt they were of poor quality, we did exclude projects that issued no final report, and, to the extent that those projects are the ones of poor quality, our sample is biased. Another factor causing similar bias stems from our treatment of received material: If the report gave a grossly inadequate description of the project in terms of the questions on the checklist, it, too, was deleted from our sample.

It should also be kept in mind that we are judging projects on the basis of the final written reports only, rather than looking at some of the other aspects, such as impact on practice. (Some of the other aspects of research do enter into the separate discussions found in earlier chapters, because our panel members were, in some instances, familiar with a piece of research and its consequences.) And finally, the report on which we base our analysis may not present an accurate account of what actually occurred during the research project.

EMPIRICAL RESULTS

To ascertain the existence of a relationship between research variables and the quality of a piece of research the following cross tabulations and regression analyses were established and analyzed. Our hope was that the analysis would confirm our earlier predictions about the influence of research-related variables upon methodological adequacy and policy utility.

Unfortunately, rater bias makes a simple review of frequency counts nearly meaningless. We therefore take two alternative approaches to the problem. First, we look at differences between overall and subcategory ratings (for example, we present the overall distribution of ratings by grantor and then review how particular grantors differ from that distribution). Second, we examine the results of regression analysis after we identify statistically similar groups of raters by use of analysis of variance.

On an overall basis 44 percent of the reports rated between one and three on methodology, while 39 percent were between four and seven, and 17 percent rated between eight and ten, the best or highest ratings. As for policy utility, 32 percent received a one-to-three rating; 42 percent received a four-to-seven rating and 26 percent were rated between eight and ten. That higher distribution for policy utility was expected, since we had asked our panel members to be cognizant of possible policy implications, even in methodologically poor reports. By doing that, we hoped to account both for the state of the art in research and for those projects to have specific implications for further research.

Grantor

As Table 14.1 indicates, the largest portion of our sample was funded by SRS. But there were enough reports from other grantors for us to believe that the trends we have isolated reflect the overall situation. Two facts stand out from Table 14.1.

First, NIMH did exceptionally well relative to our other grantors, and, second, the VA does very well on policy utility, given its low methodology ratings. (The latter was probably a result of the type of final report required by VA; the dearth of information on method in many VA reports deterred our panel members from giving high methodology ratings.

As with succeeding tabular presentations, we shall delay discussing reasons for results until the regression equations are presented.

Grantee

Given the differing incentive and constraint structures associated with grantees, we would expect them to have differential rating distributions. Our expectation is confirmed with respect to methodology, but not to a great extent regarding policy utility (see Table 14.2).

TABLE 14.1

Methodology and Policy-Utility Ratings, According to Grantor

	Methodology Rating				Policy-Utility Rating			
Grantor	1-3 (percent)	4-7 (percent)	8-10 (percent)	Total (number)	1-3 (percent)	4-7 (percent)	8-10 (percent)	Total (number)
SRS	47	37	16	313	32	42	26	315
PHS								
NIH and NIMH	42	37	21	57	26	44	30	57
NIMH	36	30	33	33	24	33	42	33
VA	36	50	14	28	28	41	31	29
Other[a]	37	42	21	71	34	42	24	71
Total	44	39	17	469[b]	32	42	26	472[b]

[a]Includes SRS-funded projects other than the basic SRS research programs, other U.S. governmental agencies, foreign governments, and private foundations. In none of those grantor types was the number large enough to justify separate tabulations.

[b]Our sample included 477 reports. In this table and the tables that follow the total number of reports varies, because not all reports could be classified according to the variable in question.

TABLE 14.2

Methodology and Policy-Utility Ratings, According to Grantee

Grantee	Methodology Rating				Policy-Utility Rating			
	1-3 (percent)	4-7 (percent)	8-10 (percent)	Total (number)	1-3 (percent)	4-7 (percent)	8-10 (percent)	Total (number)
Private rehabilitation agencies	49	38	13	135	31	40	29	136
State vocational rehabilitation agencies	44	49	7	70	31	58	11	71
Other state government agencies	46	39	16	57	32	40	28	57
Universities	34	36	30	64	23	44	33	64
Private medical institutions	39	49	13	39	39	40	28	57
VA	46	47	13	30	29	42	29	31
University medical schools	33	19	48	27	18	30	52	27
Other*	56	27	17	48	46	42	12	48
Total Sample	44	39	17	470	32	42	26	473

*Includes the following grantee types: governmentally funded medical institutions, except both university medical schools and VA; private research firms; foreign governments; schools other than universities; and others. In none of those grantee types was the number of reports large enough to justify separate tabulation.

Simply, the results show high methodological quality at universities and poor quality at state vocational-rehabilitation agencies. The most surprising result is the shift for private rehabilitation agencies from below the total sample for methodology to above the sample for policy utility. The same pattern was noted for the VA, but that result was expected: Since VA grantee and grantor are one and the same, we would guess their ratings in both categories move in the same direction and with similar magnitude.

Experimental Design

As stated earlier, we would expect the quality of design to be directly related to methodology and consequently to policy utility. One important fact should be kept in mind, however: In many cases an experimental design is not necessarily the best one for achieving a study's objectives. Hence, a lack of "true" design does not mean that the quasi-experimental or preexperimental design used was not the most appropriate for the situation. Table 14.3 gives the relationship between design and ratings. A somewhat disheartening (but not wholly unexpected) statistic is that only 52 percent of our studies reported using any experimental design. The impact of the two preferred designs—pretest/posttest control group and posttest-only control group—appears to be somewhat different. The former does better than other designs over the middle and upper ranges in both types of ratings, while the latter is much more concentrated in the middle level.

Perhaps some of the relationships between grantees and quality could be explained by the differential usage of the two preferred designs. For example, other state governmental agencies used the two designs in 42 percent of their studies, while state vocational rehabilitation agencies used the designs in 17 percent of their studies. For the former (and in both quality measures) the percentage of reports in the high or 8-to-10 category was twice as great as the corresponding percentages for the latter.

Nonexperimental Design

Another factor likely to affect the methodology ratings is the type of nonexperimental design used. Of the 228 studies using nonexperimental designs approximately 64 percent were considered demonstrations. (Again, we note the difficulties checklisters had in

TABLE 14.3

Methodology and Policy-Utility Ratings, According to Experimental Design

| Design | Methodology Rating | | | | Policy-Utility Rating | | | |
	1-3 (percent)	4-7 (percent)	8-10 (percent)	Total (number)	1-3 (percent)	4-7 (percent)	8-10 (percent)	Total (number)
One-shot case study	65	28	7	74	49	31	20	74
One-group pretest/ posttest	54	30	16	44	43	39	18	44
Pretest/posttest control group	26	48	26	42	17	50	33	42
Posttest-only control group	16	68	16	25	11	62	27	26
Other research designs	31	43	26	61	26	40	34	61
Total	43	39	17	246*	32	42	26	247*

*Includes all reports for which a research design was identified. The discrepancy between the totals in the policy-utility and the methodology ratings occurs because of one report that had no methodology rating.

TABLE 14.4

Methodology and Policy-Utility Ratings, According to Type of Nonexperimental Design

Design	Methodology Rating				Policy-Utility Rating			
	1-3 (percent)	4-7 (percent)	8-10 (percent)	Total (number)	1-3 (percent)	4-7 (percent)	8-10 (percent)	Total (number)
Demonstration	53	33	14	145	35	40	25	146
Survey	0	47	53	15	7	66	27	15
Pilot study	75	0	25	12	50	25	25	12
Descriptive or exploratory	30	56	13	16	19	50	21	16
Other*	36	51	13	39	20	54	26	39
Total	44	39	17	227	32	42	26	228

*Includes a miscellaneous group of nonexperimental design types.

distinguishing between demonstrations, one-shot case studies and
one-group pretest/posttest design.) Table 14.4 shows how nonexperimental designs fared in our ratings. The most notable feature in the
table is the high rating of surveys in terms of methodological quality
and their midrange rating for policy utility. One explanation for that
finding is the statistical orientation of the surveys, since many were
correlates of success studies.

Treatment or Independent Variables

While 95 codes were possible in this category, many of them
consisted of combinations of a crucial six or seven variables. It is
instructive to examine the variance of policy-utility ratings with
respect to some of the most often (singularly) used variables, as
well as with one significant combination. Table 14.5 gives such data.
Programs using counseling alone seemed to do well, while those
employing special education exclusively rate poorly in policy utility.
That could be due to the downward rater bias caused by our panel
member in special education.

TABLE 14.5

Policy-Utility Ratings, According to Type of Treatment

Types of Treatment	Policy-Utility Rating			
	1-3 (percent)	4-7 (percent)	8-10 (percent)	Total (number)
Counseling	12	47	41	17
Psychiatric help	27	53	20	15
Social work (home visits)	6	63	31	16
Special education	50	40	10	20
Vocational training	39	39	22	23
Counseling, vocational training, and vocational evaluation	28	55	17	18
Total	28	49	23	109

The Researchers

In 90 percent of the studies the people involved in the rehabilitation program did the research; 8 percent of the research was done by an independent party. Fifteen percent of the reports done by people involved in the program were given a poor rating of one, as compared with 3 percent of these performed by some independent party. Twenty-nine percent of the studies done by independent parties received a good rating of eight, whereas only 8 percent of the reports that were done by people involved received an eight rating. The same is true for the reports rated nine—i.e., a higher percentage of those that were done by independent parties received higher ratings than those conducted by people involved in the program. The same findings hold true for the policy-utility ratings.

Discipline

We will not go into much detail in this category for two reasons. First, it is an exercise in futility to try to classify many of the projects we saw as being from one discipline. Multidisciplinary research in rehabilitation is the rule rather than the exception. A second reason for not presenting disciplinary data with ratings is that we tried to channel reports to panel members partially based on discipline, thereby making it impossible to separate a panel member's bias from quality. While we could note the tendencies of panel members, a fine tuning of that bias is beyond our capacity at this point. As a general conclusion we note that the data do indicate that the more established, scientific disciplines (e.g., psychiatry) do better than the newer services-oriented disciplines, such as rehabilitation counseling and vocational education. That is likely due to state-of-the-art factors, as well as to the existence of possibilities for controlling variables. The policy-utility ratings show the same tendencies but to a lesser degree.

Duration

The period of time over which a project is done affects the quality of the project. (The reader should bear in mind the possible interactions between funder, funding, duration and quality). Table 14.6 presents the data for various durations for each rating category.

TABLE 14.6

Methodology and Policy-Utility Ratings, According to Duration of Project

Duration (months)	Methodology Rating				Policy-Utility Rating			
	1-3 (percent)	4-7 (percent)	8-10 (percent)	Total (number)	1-3 (percent)	4-7 (percent)	8-10 (percent)	Total (number)
6-12	44	38	18	45	49	38	13	45
13-24	38	38	23	39	23	51	26	39
25-36	41	43	15	150	28	44	28	151
37-48	50	38	12	94	34	38	28	95
49-60	43	35	22	65	31	37	32	65
61-72	57	26	17	23	35	48	17	23
73-84	62	23	15	13	46	31	23	13
Total	45	39	16	429	33	41	26	431

The durations showing the best methodology are 24 and 60 months. The dispersion is somewhat surprising. One explanation is that the two periods represent very different kinds of projects that by their nature require either a short or long period of time to be adequately done. Policy utility shows less dispersion: Only very short projects fare very poorly. That finding underscores the need for follow-up information in order to establish outcomes.

Handicap

Research on rehabilitation of persons with specific disabilities varies in quality for reasons similar to those discussed above in the discipline section. That is, some handicap areas have been subject to greater research, thereby allowing for the buildup of expertise in solving research problems. In addition, since some types of handicaps (e.g., being disadvantaged) are more susceptible to outside influences, attempts to establish control may be fruitless. The ratings for the major handicaps in our sample are presented in Table 14.7. Again, care should be taken in interpreting the data, because of correlations between handicap, panel member, and discipline and because of the small number of cases in certain handicaps. Also, the policy utility of the reports relative to handicap is no doubt related to the size and type of the population at risk. We should expect research in areas with large numbers of disabled to have broader policy utility. An examination of the data indicates that the variance in both methodology and policy utility is not inordinately large, except for the special case of medically-oriented respiratory research.

Year of Report

We expected that the methodological quality and usefulness would improve over time. The former should be due to better knowledge and information on the conduct of valid research. The latter should be a result of better identification of relevant problems. When we reviewed the data (not presented here) on that topic, no strong tendencies in either direction appeared. That is, while the research ratings in our sample did not show significant improvement over time, neither did they show significant decline.

TABLE 14.7

Methodology and Policy-Utility Ratings, According to Type of Handicap

Handicap	Methodology Rating				Policy Utility Rating			
	1-3 (percent)	4-7 (percent)	8-10 (percent)	Total (number)	1-3 (percent)	4-7 (percent)	8-10 (percent)	Total (number)
Visual impairment	52	43	7	27	33	52	15	27
Hearing impairment	57	21	21	14	57	29	14	14
Speech impairment	33	50	17	6	50	33	17	6
Mental retardation	54	34	12	97	47	26	28	98
Mental illness	46	36	18	85	33	36	31	87
Respiratory	0	25	75	8	0	12	88	8
Orthopedic	43	32	25	29	25	46	29	29
Public offender	31	44	25	36	14	56	31	36
Alcoholism	35	60	5	20	20	55	25	20
Educationally and culturally disadvantaged	38	50	12	32	25	44	31	32
Other disabled	44	39	17	116	26	56	18	116
Total	44	39	17	470	32	42	26	473

REGRESSION RESULTS

The next stage of the analysis of the data from our sample of 477 reports is the formulation and testing of a model. In such a model we seek to evaluate the relationship of certain independent variables with methodology and policy-utility ratings (our dependent variables). The model follows directly from the preceding analysis in this chapter.

One method of testing the model is regression analysis.* Using that technique we attempt to determine whether a set of variables is related to the dependent variable and whether the relationships are statistically significant. Two special problems need to be resolved before we can proceed with an analysis of our results. One is the question of rater bias, and the other is multicollinearity.

Our basic approach to the rater-bias problem was to identify groups of raters whose scores could pass an analysis of variance test. We did that in two ways: For methodology we were able to distinguish a "hard" and "easy" group of raters; for policy utility we identified a statistically coherent group of raters by dropping the hardest and easiest of raters. Therefore, our regressions were done on samples of reports reviewed by raters in each of the three groups.

When we ran the regressions with the variables listed in Equations 1, 3, and 5, we encountered significant multicollinearity. To overcome the multicollinearity problem we ran regressions (see Equations 2, 4, and 6) with fewer variables so as to eliminate much of the correlation between variables. (In the process of dropping variables from the larger equations it should be emphasized that in cases where variables in the same category remain the effect of the dropped variables can be found in the constant.) We used Haitovsky's test to test for the extent of multicollinearity in the equations. Equations 2, 4, and 6 were able to "pass" the test while Equations 1, 3, and 5 did not.

We now proceed to present the regression results and examine the relationships of variables and our two sets of ratings. A summary of results is given in Tables 14.8 (methodology ratings) and 14.9 (policy-utility ratings).

----

*For a straightforward review of the technique, see Johnston, 1972. For special consideration of the problems and strategies involved in using dummy variables see Kmenta, 1971, Chapter 11, and Chapter 11 of this book.

TABLE 14.8

Regression Results, Dependent Variable: Methodology Ratings

Variable	Equation 1 (hard raters)	Equation 2 (hard raters)	Equation 3 (easy raters)	Equation 4 (easy raters)
Constant	6.22	3.46	-2.31	1.89
Grantee type				
VA	- .69		- .89	
	(1.18)		(1.28)	
University	.24	.56	1.71	2.39
medical school	(.51)	(1.08)	(2.27)*	(3.44)*
Private medical	.18	.70	- .78	- .88
institutions	(.41)	(1.44)	(1.24)	(1.62)
University (nonmedical	.33	.77	- .12	
school)	(.92)	(2.04)*	(.19)	
State VR	- .10	.11	-1.23	
agency	(.27)	(.32)	(2.00)*	
Private rehabilitation	- .53	- .24	- .86	
center, agency, etc.	(1.75)*	(.77)	(1.79)*	
Grantor type				
SRS (Basic R&D	- .13		.48	
program	(.41)		(1.01)	
NIMH	- .55	- .09	2.57	1.85
	(1.07)	(.18)	(3.90)*	(3.05)*
VA		.36		-1.79
		(.57)		(3.18)*
Duration (years)				
1 or less	.87		.49	
	(1.86)*		(.69)	
1-2	.95		- .01	
	(1.96)*		(.01)	
2-3	.50		.98	
	(1.25)		(1.56)	
3-4	- .02		.87	
	(.04)		(1.25)	
4-5	.73		.95	
	(1.61)		(1.29)	
5-6	.59		.57	
	(.97)		(.65)	
Reasons exist due to sampling to doubt generalizability	- .57	- .86	- .74	- .64
	(2.48)*	(3.56)*	(2.23)*	(1.92)*
Experimental design and analysis				
Pretest/posttest	1.04		.19	- .08
control group	(2.58)*		(.32)	(.14)
Posttest-only	.77		-1.11*	-1.46
control group	(1.40)		(1.81)	(2.41)*
Control of 3 or more	.34		- .60	
demographic variables	(1.00)		(1.41)	
Control of 3 or more				
rehabilitation-related	- .06		1.33	1.22
variables	-(.16)		(2.54)*	(2.35)*

(continued)

(Table 14.8 continued)

Variable	Equation 1 (hard raters)	Equation 2 (hard raters)	Equation 3 (easy raters)	Equation 4 (easy raters)
Hypothesis was clearly spelled out	.84 (3.35)*	1.05 (3.95)*	.86 (2.42)*	.85 (2.28)*
Associational analysis was done	.91 (3.91)*	1.08 (4.32)*	.60 (1.71)*	.46 (1.29)
Multivariate analysis was done	1.89 (4.83)*	2.49 (6.48)*	.77 (1.46)	1.24 (2.33)*
Researcher				
People involved in the program	− .84 (2.17)*	−1.20 (3.80)*	.42 (.61)	
Unaffiliated third party	− .49 (.84)		1.45 (1.62)	
Nonexperimental design				
Demonstration	.34 (1.32)		.26 (.73)	
Follow-up	1.14 (1.55)		.19 (.18)	
Survey	− .25 (.29)		.85 (.51)	
Year of Report	− .01 (.44)		.09 (1.94)*	.04 (1.03)
Adjusted funding for project	.16 (2.07)*		.02 (.11)	
Panel member				
Rater 6	− .95 (1.27)			
Rater 2	−2.64 (3.70)*			
Rater 3	−3.21 (4.43)*			
Rater 9			.07 (.09)	
Rater 5			−1.73 (2.25)*	
Rater 10			− .42 (.56)	
Rater 7			1.28 (1.88)*	
Rater 1			−1.67 (2.07)*	
Summary statistics				
R^2	.5498	.4177	.3435	.2482
F	11.3062	17.1377	4.1554	6.64
Haitovsky's test	.01647	108.41147	.01547	117.83311
Degrees of freedom for Haitovsky's test	528	78	595	78

Note: The coefficients for each equation are as listed with t values in parentheses. An asterisk indicates that the variable was significant at the 95-percent confidence level for a one-tailed t-test.

TABLE 14.9

Regression Results, Dependent Variable: Policy-Utility Ratings

Variable	Equation 5	Equation 6
Constant	3.39	2.90
Grantee type		
University medical school	.65	
	(.89)	
Private medical institution	- .53	
	(.85)	
University (nonmedical school)	.78	
	(1.35)	
State VR agency	- .09	- .55
	(.16)	(1.44)
Private rehabilitation center,	- .28	- .62
agency, etc.	(.52)	(1.96)*
State agency (non-VR)	.31	
	(.53)	
Grantor type		
SRS (Basic R&D program)	.34	.29
	(.88)	(.86)
NIMH	.88	.79
	(1.63)	(1.57)
State government or agency		-1.58
		(2.10)*
VA	- .39	
	(.58)	
Reasons exist due to sampling to	- .79	- .86
doubt generalizability	(2.85)*	(3.22)*
Experimental design and analysis		
Pretest/posttest control group	.87	.82
	(1.85)*	(1.85)*
Posttest-only control group	.30	
	(.57)	
Associational analysis was done	.78	.85
	(2.73)*	(3.15)*
Multivariate analysis was done	1.66	1.75
	(3.76)*	(4.33)*
Report not understandable	- .83	
	(1.38)	
Nonexperimental design		
Pilot	.99	
	(.91)	
Demonstration	- .04	
	(.11)	
Follow-up	.96	
	(1.22)	
Survey	.17	
	(.24)	

(continued)

(Table 14.9 continued)

Variable	Equation 5	Equation 6
Dependent variable		
Employment status was included	- .48	
	(1.60)	
Self-concept was included	- .22	
	(.29)	
Independent living was included	- .01	
	(.01)	
Year of Report	.03	.03
	(.68)	(.97)
Research not capable of being replicated	- .43	
	(.62)	
Summary statistics		
R^2	.1485	.1550
F	3.4641	7.2168
Haitovsky's tests	9.05573	188.20595
Degrees of freedom for Haitovsky's test	300	55

Note: The coefficients for each equation are listed with t values in parentheses. An asterisk indicates that the variable was significant at the 95-percent confidence level for a one-tailed t-test.

Grantee

Only a few grantees had any significant effect on either of our
ratings. Research done at private rehabilitation centers, agencies,
and so on, tended to have a negative impact on policy utility, while
research at universities was generally associated with good methodology. The former result was not entirely expected. One possible
reason for the rehabilitation-agency-policy-utility relationship is
the poor methodology associated with research done by the agencies.
The university result was expected due to the nature of our judgment
criteria and existing academic research standards.

Grantor

The four major grantors all showed varying effects on the
ratings. SRS had no significant impact on either rating; state government or agency as a grantor was negatively associated with policy
utility; NIMH was significant and positive in relation to methodology
for the easy-rater sample, while having a negative but not significant
effect on methodology for the hard-rater sample; VA had a significant
and negative effect on methodology rating for the easy raters and no
significant effect for the other raters. The last result was not unexpected, given the relationship between VA as grantee and grantor
and our earlier tabular analysis. The fact that a state government
or agency may have a negative effect on policy utility could be explained by the type of projects they fund. For example, those grantors
may be funding previously reviewed areas through their concern for
providing adequate services, thereby limiting the project's policy
utility, as we have defined it. Other results are likely due to proposal design and reporting requirements.

Duration

The optimal length of time over which a project should run will
vary depending upon a number of related variables, such as type of
research, researchers, and so on. As in the tabular section, no
real conclusions about optimal duration could be reached.

Design Analysis

The set of variables relating to sampling, design, and statistical analysis were the most important ones in explaining both sets of ratings. As expected, when sampling problems arose, leading to questions about a project's generalizability, both methodology and policy-utility ratings were significantly and negatively effected.

We also tested the impact of the two preferred experimental designs. For policy utility, the effect of using the pretest/posttest experimental design was positive and significant. A somewhat surprising result was the significant and negative effect of the posttest-only control-group design on methodology for the easy-rater sample. The only explanation we can offer is the inconsistency of standards that may exist for that sample. The methodology ratings of the sample were not affected by the use of the pretest/posttest control-group design. That was not the case for the hard-rater sample, whose ratings were positively affected by the design. (That variable was not included in Equation 2 because its addition led to multicollinearity difficulties.)

Another important variable with regard to methodology ratings was the clarity with which hypotheses were formulated and stated. That variable had a positive and significant impact. Our panel members seemed to feel that if a researcher was clear in intent, it could be considered a plus in evaluating methodological design.

The use of statistical analysis also had a positive and significant effect for both ratings. The more sophisticated methods, as indicated in the multivariate analysis variable, had the greater impact. (The nature of much rehabilitation research might require multivariate analysis; it is not inherently superior to univariate techniques.) Such broad confirmation of what was expected should not be regarded lightly. The need for quality statistical analysis in research seems to be critical if results are to be correctly interpreted.

It was felt that nonexperimental designs would move closely with policy utility, but no such relationship was indicated in Equation 5. A similar result was associated with various dependent variables that we included in the policy-utility equation.

Other Variables

For the hard-rater sample we found that when research was done by those involved in the program, the methodology rating was

negatively affected. That was a confirmation of our tabular analysis
and could serve as a guide to grantors in expending research funds.

It appears evident that the year in which a project was completed
could serve as a proxy for current ideas. In that context one could
expect more recent projects to have greater policy utility. That conclusion was not confirmed by the data. One reason is that we asked
panel members to rate reports with an eye toward the state of the
art. Doing that would counteract the previously stated effect of
current ideas.

As for funding, results again were inconclusive. There did
appear to be some tendency in the hard-rater sample for funding to
move in the same direction as methodology. The impact of that
variable on research outcome measures deserved further, more
specific, statistical analysis.

SUMMARY AND CONCLUSIONS

In this chapter we have summarized, reviewed, and analyzed
the data collected during our project. We have set forth some ideas
and theories about the relationship between research variables and
outcome measures. It is important to emphasize that what we have
uncovered and confirmed is based on a sample of projects chosen on
the limited criteria set forth in Chapter 1. Also, our results are
clearly a function of the checklist we used and of the ideas and biases
of the faculty members we chose to judge rehabilitation research.
Other people with a different set of reports on rehabilitation research
might very well find varying results. Yet, given these limitations
and caveats, we feel quite confident in making some general conclusions on the subject of the methodology and policy usefulness of
research in those areas of rehabilitation for which we have gathered
reports.

Were one concerned with spending funds to obtain methodologically acceptable research it would appear necessary to consider a
number of alternative aspects of research. (Again, as we did in
Chapter 1, we should note that methodological adequacy and policy
utility are not always the goals of research. For research with
different goals our project is of limited usefulness as regards its
recommendations.) The people given the task of undertaking research
should be generally familiar with the tools of statistical analysis and
experimental design. They should have no special concern about the
successful conclusion of a project or the confirming of research
hypotheses. Moreover, they should be aware that they will be judged
on the quality of their evaluation and not on the success or failure of a
project.

The grantor through which research funds are to be funneled should be one with some proposal-review system established to insure that the researcher uses the appropriate methodological criteria. When this structure exists, a project will be on the correct track for adequate methodology from the earliest stages.

One of the critical areas of research that needs to be emphasized is that of sampling procedures. It is important that research samples be chosen in such a manner that any results of the project be generalizable to some larger population.

Another important aspect of a research project is the experimental design. While the correct design depends on the hypothesis and project under study, some design is necessary to be able to identify the true effects of the treatment variables. Without adequate design the results of a project are open to question. In general the methodological adequacy of the research will be weakened. Similar arguments are apropos in the case of statistical analysis.

As regards achieving policy utility, a research project should be most concerned with methodology. The two outcomes measures are clearly associated, with the former being limited by weaknesses in the latter. Many of the same variables were significant in the policy-utility and methodology equations. Other factors we felt to be important in policy utility were the size of the population at risk and the implications of a project for further research. While we were unable to measure the variables extensively, we feel they cannot be ignored by grantors seeking policy usefulness in their funded projects.

An area of further research of the sort reported here is in the estimation of optimal duration and the impact of funding on quality of research. For example, do certain types of projects need specific, varying periods of time to be acceptable methodologically or useful as policy? Does the amount of project funding have a significant impact on research quality?

The results discussed above are not revolutionary. They generally reconfirm earlier expectations and previously stated standards. Our project can serve its greatest purpose as a platform from which to urge the reform of the structure and character of research.

REFERENCES

Bernstein, I., Rieker, P., and Freeman, H. A Review of Evaluation Research: The State of the Art Methodological Practice, and Dissemination of Research Findings. New York: Russell Sage Foundation, 1973.

Campbell, D., and Stanley, J. Experimental and Quasi-Experimental
     Designs for Research. Chicago: Rand McNally, 1966.

DeGeyndt, W. Methodological Adequacy of Federal R&D Projects.
     Minneapolis, Minn.: Minnesota Systems Research, Inc.,
     1973.

Johnston, J. Econometric Methods. New York: McGraw-Hill, 1972.

Kmenta, J. Elements of Econometrics. New York: Macmillan, 1971.

Muthard, J., Wells, S., and Crocker, L. Research Applied to Policy
     and Practice: A Method for Assessing the Impact of Selected
     Research and Demonstration Projects. unpublished, Regional
     Rehabilitation Research Institute, University of Florida, Miami,
     Fla., 1973.

Rivlin, A. Systematic Thinking for Social Action. Washington, D.C.:
     The Brookings Institution, 1971.

Rossi, P., and Williams, W., eds. Evaluating Social Action Pro-
     grams Theory, Practice, and Politics. New York: Seminar
     Press, 1972.

Evaluation of what in many cases was evaluation research is a sensitive business. Our purpose, to identify quality research and examine its implications for rehabilitation practice, puts us in the position of indicating departures from adequate research methodology. Taking a role such as this required us to account for a myriad of variables inherent in the field of rehabilitation leading to problems in research and evaluation design. The separate difficulties of doing research in rehabilitation and evaluation become compounded when they are combined.

Examples of those difficulties and their impact on the final product appear throughout this book. We intend in this concluding chapter to review how these difficulties impinge on the methodological quality and policy utility of the research in our sample. Finally, we plan to propose some recommendations for ways to rectify or bypass the problems or to produce adequate research and evaluation within the constraints they create.

METHODOLOGY

Only a small percentage of the reports reviewed by our panel members were of sufficient methodological quality to be rated at the upper end of our scale. The explanation of that result depends on more than the kinds of problems discussed above (and in detail below). A certain carelessness with regard to research design and data collection was apparent in a number of reports. In many cases those conducting the project either lacked the support or capability to design their work correctly or felt no need to justify their approach.*

The existence of a problem of that type has its origins with grantors as much as with grantees. Failure on the part of the grantor to require preprogram information on design and methodology or to provide sufficient funds or researchers to conduct the research or evaluation often manifested itself in a poor outcome. When a final report on a research project contains only descriptive material based on "impressions," a lack of control or the nonexistence of any type of incentives or disincentives is a likely cause. It is the grantor who must bear the responsibility for such failure.

An additional reason for the poor methodology ratings is that as research proceeds, more complex matters come into play. For example, public awareness that, in order to serve as a control group, some may have to be deprived of a service in the present, has created political resistence to a necessary aspect of many research designs. The innumerable outside factors operating on project participants makes identification of the independent variables truly difficult. The recognition that many outcome measures are too simplistic to be useful has also added to the problems of achieving adequate methodological design and procedure. Those factors have had growing influence over time, thereby·increasing the difficulty involved in research design.

Other aspects of research convergent with poor methodology were also noted by our panel members. Two of the variables in particular lack the excuse of changing expectations over time. One such example related to outcome measurement is follow-up design and analysis. The necessity of follow-ups structured so as to measure the "strength" of an achieved outcome has been reaffirmed by all earlier authors. Again and again, the failure to incorporate the time period following rehabilitation explicitly was cited as a critical item in the rating judgment. A second—and perhaps less acceptable— factor in poor methodology is the inadequate and incorrect use of statistical techniques and measures. Those tools are available and can readily be applied to aid in the interpretation of research findings.

In sum, we have seen through the sample of reports analyzed in our project that rehabilitation research and evaluation have yet

---

*A reason for the second possibility has been hinted at by a number of chapter authors. They note the tendency for many projects to reenact old and existing approaches. While to some extent such replication is necessary, it should not serve as a means to avoid doing a methodologically correct study.

to achieve a consistently good methodological approach. Counterexamples were numerous enough to be encouraging. Chapter 14 has shown those grantees and grantors that have been most successful in the past. The characteristics of those researchers and funders that we feel are critical to methodological quality will be incorporated in our recommendations below. Other aspects of research that were correlated with methodological quality, such as experimental design, statistical analysis, follow-up, and so on, will also be a part of our suggestions for the future. Before making such ideas a part of a program for rehabilitation research, we will discuss the other standard we used to judge rehabilitation research: policy utility.

POLICY UTILITY

Our review has uncovered no new paradigm in the rehabilitation of the handicapped. No one method or technique has been shown to be consistently better than another. For a different people different approaches work. No one treatment can serve as the basis or guideline along which all rehabilitation should proceed. Yet certain techniques when used on particular types of people have been shown to be effective. The proven effectiveness of methods for rehabilitation is what we have identified as policy utility.

In judging the policy utility of a research project, particular variables were shown to be of major significance. First and foremost was the need for a project and evaluation to be methodologically sound. Failure to meet that criterion usually meant failure to have much usefulness for policy.

Another aspect of a project that came to the fore in assessing a project's usefulness for policy was the possible returns relative to costs. Many of our reviewers stressed the need to measure program efficiency. As has been pointed out elsewhere, that task involves the estimation and measurement of costs and benefits. In rehabilitation practice that is not an easy task; in rehabilitation research it is very nearly impossible on a preproject basis. Yet some measures of the likely research costs and chances of success and effective implementation are needed. The identification of variables significantly related to research outcome should be given high priority. We feel the analysis in this book, especially in Chapter 14, moves us well along toward our goal. When such research measures are tested and perfected, grantors will be in a much better position to choose grantees and projects most likely to contribute to policy in the rehabilitation field.

Some of the other critical variables in the relationship between research and policy are program feasibility, population of likely beneficiaries, and the relationship between researchers and practitioners. Regarding feasibility, if the program, technique, or treatment being tested fails to meet acceptable standards of ethical, moral, or organizational feasibility, its implementation will be stymied. While recognition of that aspect of policy utility limits the options of the researcher such an awareness in the preproject period will help grantors avoid funding projects likely to have only an insignificant policy impact.

One important recent development related to the feasibility of wide-scale implementation of certain research results is neighborhood or community opposition. Projects that confirm the effectiveness of halfway houses or group homes generally imply the introduction of outsiders into a neighborhood. That has generated fear, and the resulting opposition has held up introduction of facilities whose success in many cases has been indicated by research. That result suggests two possibilities: One is to recognize the existence of such opposition and to attempt to overcome it by reasoned discussion or adjustment in program design; a second possibility is to require researchers to incorporate such feasibility constraints into their analysis.

The total number of people subject to the possible uses of research output will certainly help determine how useful a project will be. If the population-at-risk is small, there is likely to be less policy utility (in a global sense) associated with a project related to their limitations. On the other hand, if the population-at-risk is large, even small gains attained through research could have a large impact on our measure of usefulness.

Finally, researchers must take into account the needs of practitioners. What a practitioner is willing to incorporate in a rehabilitation program can serve as a partial guideline to researchers in the development, design, and process of their project. In the reverse direction practitioners should remain open to methods, techniques, and treatments whose effectiveness has been established through vigorous research activities.

RESEARCHERS AND PRACTITIONERS

The relationships between researchers and practitioners are more complex than indicated by the preceding paragraph, and the nature of the relationships becomes particularly important in the critical area of the selection of research topics and the transmission and utilization of research results. To get at the heart of the matter we need to understand the goals of both researchers and practitioners, as well as the constraints under which each group works.

Researchers have as their goal the design, management, and analysis of a project that hopefully will provide knowledge to aid in the rehabilitation of the handicapped. In that context researchers possess enormous leeway. For example, the identification of a research issue can arise out of cooperation with practitioners or evolve from the researcher's own estimates of the needs of the rehabilitation program. The researcher also has a wide choice in the methodological aspects of a project. He can choose to follow accepted design and analysis criteria strictly, or he can structure the project to achieve certain ends and report only what he wishes. The former is likely to be less understandable to the practitioner, and the latter to be invalid from a scientific standpoint.

Practitioners seek to use techniques that achieve the most significant results for clients. The needs of practitioners are thus directly derived from the types of clients they see. To some extent, then, researchable issues are given to, and not chosen by, the practitioners. Researchers face a different situation, unencumbered by such constraints. Thus, a list of research issues constructed by each would probably be only partially correlated.

If one accepts the scenario above, the logical conclusion or suggestion that emerges is the requiring of greater preproject collaboration between researchers and practitioners. From the welter of conflicting ideas should come a consensus on the problems that should be studied, analyzed, and solved. Practitioners' ideas probably deserve greater weight in arriving at such a consensus, since it is they who can best identify their clients' needs. Researchers must be involved on two levels: One is the translation of practitioners' needs into researchable questions; the other is the review of researcher insights on ideas and issues, possibly outside the ken of practitioners. Both roles are important, and both must be taken into account.

Two additional topics related to the roles of practitioners and researchers are the methodology and utilization of research. Design and reporting of research are critical to the final uses made of a project's results. The utilization of research depends not only on the relevancy of the topic to the needs of practitioners but also on the understanding that practitioners have about what was done.

Practitioners may show little interest in methodological questions, but it is essential that they not rely on results derived from projects that have not firmly established their hypothesis due to methodological inadequacies. Intuition may be a better guide. On the other hand, scientifically established research results couched in technical jargon may be equally useless. Obviously, if results are to be utilized, they must be communicated to the practitioners working in the field.

Several possible solutions to the problem can be suggested. First, researchers could be encouraged to produce two reports, one stressing methodology and design and the other concentrating on results and their implications. Conversely, some practitioners could be encouraged to become better acquainted with methodological criteria and techniques. That possibility would be a significant step in creating a constituency that demands, interprets, and utilizes, methodologically correct research.

Other methods for establishing such a constituency should be encouraged. The establishment of a rehabilitation journal in which research is reported and critically reviewed could be a step in the right direction. A section of that journal might contain a review by practitioners on the implications of research for practice. A second suggestion along those lines would be an increase in the use of the research-utilization specialists now employed in several state agencies. We envision their role as similar to that served by a journal—i.e., to review critically, evaluate, interpret, and suggest uses for research results. The development of a research constituency in rehabilitation would increase freedom for researchers to pursue scientific goals and at the same time increase the practitioners' store of interpretable and usable knowledge.

IMPROVING THE QUALITY OF RESEARCH

A series of recommendations regarding the future direction of research in rehabilitation appears in each of the previous chapters. There is no need for us to reiterate them here. Rather, we shall recommend changes in the review, administration, and conduct of research grants. Our proposals have as their basis an attempt to make research more methodologically complete while maintaining the close (and necessary) ties with reality and the needs of those who are directly involved in the practice of rehabilitation. The task is not easy. It calls for changes in the ways in which many things have previously been done. Yet, if we are to get a research output commensurate with the inputs, such a reorientation is a necessary condition.

One of the most striking tendencies we noted was the close relationship between poor-quality research and internal conduct of the evaluation. When those responsible for the operation of the program were also given responsibility for research design and evaluation, an imperfect product was the likely output. A number of reasons may account for that result. One explanation might be the bias associated with self-evaluation. A second possibility is an inability or unwillingness on the part of the people involved to design and evaluate research, in part because they remain unconvinced that the quality of the research has any relationship to the usefulness of outcomes. Another associated explanation is that no pressure or request for quality research design came from the grantor. Also perhaps the funds available were not large enough to do both the experiment desired and an accurate evaluation.

Those causes suggest a number of alternatives in the direction and organization of research. Perhaps most important is the need for guidance and the provision of incentives. The grantor should bear immediate responsibility for providing these. The use of peer review and a possible alternative has been amply discussed by Noble (1974).* As a minimum, some form of thorough ex ante review should be carried out. Such a review should emphasize the requirements of experimental design and the constraints inspired by the world in which practitioners live. In addition, some formalized ex post review should be conducted either by an impartial internal agency staff or a panel recruited from outside the agency.

The review serves two major purposes. First, the results should be used as a partial basis for a future allocation of research with preference for those rating high in methodology and policy utility.† Second, the data collected through such a review procedure could serve as a basis for a complete determination of variables most significantly related to suggested outcome measures. Identifying those variables would provide a means to improve the efficiency of the allocation of future funds.

Along with (or instead of) tighter agency direction as prescribed above, a separation of the service aspects of the program from research and evaluation of R&D seems necessary. Separation of those aspects of a project should result in an improvement in experimental design and data analysis, as well as in the attainment of a higher degree of scientific integrity in the presentation of results. But as with the practitioner-researcher problem, the early establishment of a working relationship between researcher and evaluator is essential. When adequate coordination occurs early and is maintained, both the project director and research evaluator are likely to prosper through trades each must make to meet the demands of the other.

------

*Noble, J.H., Jr., "Peer Review: Quality Control of Applied Social Research." Science 185 (September 13, 1974), pp. 916-921.

†An implicit assumption here is that the agency is concerned with methodological adequacy and usefulness. If for some reason those are not primary R&D goals, our suggestions would require substantial adjustments.

The proposed guidelines for ex ante and ex post review and independence can help in achieving methodological quality, but they lack the strength to guarantee policy utility. A few suggestions along those lines have been culled from the chapters submitted by panel members and are expanded upon below.

Many projects failed to formulate a firm theoretical construct on which to base their research. In cases of that sort, hypotheses are not likely to be clearly specified and in fact may go unstated. A floating goal structure, or the complete absence of an objective function, can lead to numerous evaluation difficulties. Any project can be deemed successful, if the program managers are allowed to formulate their intentions after the results are determined. Before receiving funding, grantees should be required to emphasize their cause-and-effect linkages so that outcome measures and policy implications can be established.

Outcome measures have to be considered in the context of hypothesis formulation. Many of the reports we reviewed failed to provide an adequate measure of success. In too many instances, success measurement was finalized at the end of an experiment with no subsequent follow-up. Obviously, the "staying power" of a rehabilitation program outweighs its immediate impact. For example, if placement in a labor-market situation were our only criterion of success, uncertainty over the ultimate and true effectiveness of a program will linger. Perhaps what is needed is some form of multiple criteria. An index might be constructed based on such variables as the length of stay in a position, movement up (or down) the job ladder, possible client achievement in the absence of rehabilitation, overall physical and mental status of the individual, and so on.

One aspect of rehabilitation programs that appeared to rate consistently high with our panel members was the need for projects to incorporate a real-world element into their design. For example, the actual program can take place in such an environment, or perhaps some transitional component can be built into the design. Of major consequence in this regard is the obvious necessity to overcome the negative attitudes toward the handicapped held by many would-be employers and fellow employees.

SUMMARY

Feasible solutions have been shown to exist for the problems discussed at the opening of this chapter. Those problems are not intractable. A number of options are open to both the grantee and grantor to improve methodological adequacy and policy utility. What is critically needed is the determination to get on with perfecting a research-grant structure and improving the workings of the market for the supply and demand of knowledge on rehabilitation.

The seemingly constant state of flux in the grant structure in recent years has hindered the achievement of quality research. What is required is a simple, straightforward, and clearly designed format for proposal review and selection.* A system along those lines would involve a decision on research issues, a proposal review based on compliance with stated methodological criteria and policy objectives, and a final review authority. The first two stages in the process are not easy, but they lie at the crux of what is at issue, for if the government has certain objectives about how and what is to be studied, the choice of proposals should be based upon the potential of the proposed projects for meeting those goals. With qualified personnel, who can see the connections between objectives and proposed projects conducting the review process, we shall be able to make the best use of funds allocated to rehabilitation research.

A structure along the lines of that prescribed above could go a long way towards the improvement of research. Combined with a willingness on the part of researchers and evaluators to incorporate and improve the tools of design and evaluation, an approach of that type could prove a significant addition to the search for knowledge regarding the most effective means to rehabilitate the handicapped.

The importance of producing research (and, thus, supplying knowledge) that has a methodological quality allowing for generalization and replication and a high degree of policy utility resulting from a responsible reading of the demands of practitioners can hardly be overstated. As policy makers come more and more to the realization that not to rehabilitate someone involves large human and economic costs, the demand for knowledge about the rehabilitation process will grow. A research program (correctly planned, designed, and executed) is the major step in providing a supply of knowledge to meet this demand.

---

*Plans and programs, such as those in "Research and Demonstration Strategy, Fiscal Year 1975" by the Rehabilitation Services Administration (RSA), appear to be on the right path. The 1975 plans are only the most recent manifestation of a procedure that has been undertaken since 1972.

SUMMARY OF CHECKLIST INFORMATION

Below is a summary of information we attempted to collect on the checklist for each report. The actual 15-page questionnaire is not replicated here for reasons of space. Copies of the checklist may be obtained from the Disability and Health Economics Research Section, Rutgers University. A checklist was filled out for each of the 477 reports in our sample.

General Information

Title of report, author(s), affiliation, grantee, grantor, description, hypothesis, discipline, subject matter, handicap, and start and completion of project.

Sampling Information

Description of the sample and how it was selected, sample size, doubts about generalizability due to a) sample size and/or b) representativeness and/or c) procedures for drawing sample.

Data Gathering

Data sources (questionnaires, tests, interviews, and so on) treatment of nonresponses, refusals, and/or dropouts (affect on results).

Methodology and Data Analysis

Type of design (experimental-nonexperimental, with further breakdown within each group), follow-up (including description and results where applicable), research variables (treatment and outcome variables and how they were operationalized and/or measured), independent variables (including demographic, rehabilitation-related, and socioeconomic variables and data on the level of analysis, i.e., considered, analyzed or controlled), clarity and testability of hypothesis, statistical procedures, i.e., descriptive statistics (means, medians, percentages, and so on), associational analysis (chi-square, Z, F or t test), or multivariate analysis (multiple regression, analysis of variance, factor analysis).

Results

Results and conclusions of the project, pertinent information on uncontrolled external influences or internal program characteristics.

Policy Utility

Who did the research (independent or someone involved in program operation), general usability of the project or procedure, doubts or difficulties in putting results to use, usefulness to rehabilitation (as empirical findings, conceptual contribution, and/or methods), accessibility and manipulability of independent variables for practitioners, likely effect of outcome due to independent variables, ethical, economic, and organizational feasibility of using the variables in practice, conflicts with other results.

Ratings

Methodology-data analysis rating, policy-utility rating.

The project was begun by the Disability and Health Economics Research Section (DHER) under the acting directorship of Professor William G. Johnson, who was responsible for its administration in its beginning stages. Working with him at the time was Edward H. Murphy and Valerie Englander. Ms. Englander stayed with the project from the beginning until its conclusion. She began the initial search for rehabilitation literature, set up the original checklisting system, and participated in the beginning analysis. Her contributions to the project continued throughout its term, both at the administrative level and in an analytical capacity. She has been responsible for quality factor analysis and the analysis of trends in rehabilitation research.

Jack Oldham, coauthor of Chapter 12, helped develop the checklist and to recruit and train people to fill them out.

Jeffrey Rubin joined the project in October 1973. He has been responsible for the day-to-day management of the project and for liaison with the students who did the checklisting and the faculty members who wrote the individual chapters. Mr. Rubin has also taken on the chief burden of editing the final manuscript and bringing the project together. He has been responsible for the introductory and cost-benefit chapters.

John D. Worrall has been the statistical consultant and has worked on several aspects of the project. He is responsible for the chapter on the correlates of success.

DHER had the benefit of an advisory panel that met with staff in the beginning phases of this project. In addition to members who contributed chapters, the panel consisted of:

John M. Atthowe, Jr., Professor of Psychology, New Jersey College of Medicine and Dentistry

Roger W. Birnbaum, Executive Director, Rutgers Community Health Plan

Miriam G. Dinerman, Professor of Social Work, Rutgers College

Joseph J. Seneca, Chairman, Department of Economics, Rutgers College

Norman Sprague, Project Director, Human Resources Center

Richard Sullivan, Medical Director, Kessler Institute for Rehabilitation

Michael K. Taussig, Professor of Economics, Rutgers College

Bruce W. Tuckman, Professor, Vocational Education, Rutgers College

Susan Viddish kept track of the research reports and competently coordinated these reports with checklists.

Ruth Agans, DHER's lead applications programmer, was responsible for the programming and computer analysis for the project.

Nina Shoehalter did much of the editorial work, helping to make intelligible and a bit more uniform the contributions of the group that provided inputs into the final reports.

The typing of the many versions of the report fell to Bernadette Hobbs and Valerie LaPorte, all capably supervised and coordinated by Laura Ford.

Susan Wheeler, Catherine Yoncheff, and Barbara Bullock spent long hours to compile the index.

MONROE BERKOWITZ is Professor of Economics at Rutgers College and the Graduate School at Rutgers University. His main fields of interest are the economics of disability and social welfare.

Mr. Berkowitz has edited volumes on rehabilitation and has served as consultant to the World Health Organization, the U.S. Social Security Administration, the Council of Economic Advisers, the National Cancer Institute, and rehabilitation and workers' compensation agencies in several states. He was an active consultant to the President's Commission on State Workmen's Compensation Laws and edited their three-volume Supplemental Studies. He has been designated as a charter Mary E. Switzer Memorial Fellow for 1975 by the National Rehabilitation Association.

His articles and reviews have appeared in the National Rehabilitation Journal, Rehabilitation Literature, Industrial Gerontology, the Industrial and Labor Relations Review, and the Journal of Human Resources.

Mr. Berkowitz holds a B.A. degree from Ohio University and M.A. and Ph.D. degrees from Columbia University.

VALERIE ENGLANDER is a research associate in the Disability and Health Economics Research Section of the Bureau of Economic Research at Rutgers University. She has a B.A. in mathematics from Upsala College and an M.A. and Ph.D. in economics from Rutgers University. Her current research involves the development of a model data system for workers' compensation.

JEFFREY RUBIN is a research associate at DHER and an instructor in the Department of Economics of Rutgers College. Mr. Rubin received an A.B. in mathematics from Rutgers College and is concluding work on his Ph.D. in economics at Duke University. Mr. Rubin's current research is in financing higher education and the evaluation of the structure and functions of disability programs.

JOHN D. WORRALL is the assistant director at DHER. He has received a B.A. and M.A. in Economics from Rutgers University and is currently concluding work on his Ph.D. Mr. Worrall's research is in the general area of the rehabilitation of the disabled, with a special emphasis on the use of benefit-cost analysis as an evaluation methodology.

As identified in the text, certain of the chapters were written by faculty members and other specialists with backgrounds in social work, sociology, psychology and vocational and special education. The current position of the authors is given in the report. They consist mainly of Rutgers University faculty and their graduate students, although two are from nearby schools.

ACCOUNTABILITY IN HEALTH FACILITIES:
Harry I. Greenfield

THE EFFECTIVENESS OF CORRECTIONAL
TREATMENT: A Survey of Treatment Evaluation
Studies
Douglas Lipton, Robert Martinson
and Judith Wilks

CHANGING THE MEDICAL CARE SYSTEM: A
Controlled Experiment in Comprehensive Care
Leon S. Robertson, John Kosa,
Margaret C. Heagarty, Robert J.
Haggerty, and Joel J. Alpert
Foreword by Charles A. Janeway

SOCIAL SCIENCE AND PUBLIC POLICY IN THE
UNITED STATES
Irving Louis Horowitz and
James Everett Katz